Alzheimer's Disease

A Holistic Approach

D1308095

Alzheimer's Disease
A Holistic Approach

Michelle Deetken, PhD

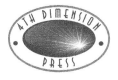

4th Dimension Press ■ Virginia Beach ■ Virginia

4th Dimension Press
215 67th Street
Virginia Beach, VA 23451-2061

ISBN 13: 978-0-87604-735-4

Cover design by Christine Fulcher

Contents

Acknowledgments

I dedicate this book to my loving husband for having the utmost patience with me during the lengthy time it took me to finish this important project. Knowingly and unknowingly, he has been my "test pilot" during our many years of residing together in health and happiness. I also want to thank my mother Reba and my uncles Jim and Ron, who are the reasons why I wrote this book. I hope they continue to live a healthy and happy life that is full of wonderful memories. I am also very grateful to the A.R.E. for carrying on the work and legacy of Edgar Cayce.

~

Introduction

I wrote this book to empower people to take control of their own health. Even though we are aging, certain lifestyle changes can and will improve our nutritional, environmental, and emotional well-being.

There are many simple things that we can do to improve the overall health of our bodies. At present, it can be stated with certainty that the whole body is affected by its nutritional status. As demonstrated by many studies, dietary factors play major roles in determining whether the brain ages successfully or declines as a result of neurodegenerative disorders. Thus, the rewards of consistently eating a nutritious diet are definitely worthwhile. With this book, I hope to show how easy it is to make lifestyle changes that will allow us to reap the rewards of growing old gracefully.

The information in the readings of Edgar Cayce inspired me to change my life for the better by making numerous small changes not only for my body's physical health but also for my mental and spiritual health. The amazing insights of the Cayce readings and the latest medical research on Alzheimer's disease and inflammation compelled me to write this book.

My introduction to Edgar Cayce happened in 1982 when I

read Jess Stearn's book, *Edgar Cayce: The Sleeping Prophet*. I signed up as an A.R.E. member halfway through the book and have been studying the Cayce readings ever since. Edgar Cayce is considered the Father of Holistic Medicine, and his work inspired me to achieve a PhD in Holistic Nutrition.

The Edgar Cayce readings have always fascinated me because they were meant to engage our very being, or essence, on so many levels. His language requires concentration to read and understand what he was trying to convey on those different levels. The first sets of levels were personal, universal, and metaphysical. Within those he incorporated more levels: the spirit, the mind, and the physical. As I have matured, I have noticed that the same reading or passage that I read in previous years will give me a new meaning—as though I were reading it for the first time. I believe that an important part of sustaining a healthy brain is learning to understand various aspects of our lives on a completely new level. Allowing our perceptions to change helps our brains to stay fit.

Following are some of the Cayce "gems" that have helped me on different levels. The numbers after a quote relate to the person who received the reading and the number of readings that the person received. Edgar Cayce's readings were organized this way because he gave over 14,000 readings, and these assigned numbers protected the person's identity. The numbered readings allowed anyone to reference a reading for research—hence the name of the organization, the Association for Research and Enlightenment (A.R.E.).

Here are some of my favorite quotes:

> . . . But hold to the ideal. Choose aright, and then go straight ahead; knowing that the Lord helps those who help themselves *provided* their purposes are not of a selfish or egotistical nature.   2437-1

The "ideal" is central to Edgar Cayce's philosophy. It is your guiding light in this world. My personal ideal is the Golden Rule: "Do unto others as you would have them to do unto you." My other ideal, which incorporates my main outlook on life, is "Celebrate the work of the Creative Spirit through nature." Everyone's ideal will be different and in tune with his or her unique life.

. . . For the only sin of man is *selfishness!*

(Q) How may it be overcome?

(A) Just as has been given; showing mercy, showing grace, showing peace, long-suffering, brotherly love, kindness — even under the most *trying* circumstances . . .   987-4

Cayce called these attributes the "fruits of the Spirit." He states repeatedly in his readings that "Mind is the Builder" and that the fruits of the Spirit are love, peace, patience (long–suffering), kindness, gentleness, mercy, and grace.

. . . but learn to use *well* that *had* in hand, then *more* may be *given* thee. Remember the talents!   2254-1

(Q) How can people avoid aging in appearance?

(A) The *mind!*   1947-4

This idea is intriguing on so many levels!

And finally, I like this quote from the readings:

Let not thy heart be troubled; ye believe in God, believe also in Him—who is able to quicken the life as it flows through thy body, thy mind, thy soul, to a full regeneration in the material world, then hope in the mental, then truth in the spiritual . . .   2448-2

~

My Grandfather's Story

"It's like a maze in here," he grumbled to himself as he wandered around the huge and dreary hospital. He knew Betty must be somewhere in one of the rooms. Why else would he be here since he was not the one wearing the hospital gown! He kept looking into every room, but he did not recognize a soul.

He knew his memory was going, but he thought, "Hell, I know what my wife looks like!" Did he somehow wind up on the wrong floor? "Darn memory," he thought, now starting to panic just a little. Next room, still no Betty. "Maybe I am here for my grandson," he theorized, "I did pass by some rooms with children in them."

He stops a nurse and asks her if he is on the children's floor. She told him that the children's ward was in another wing and ran off in a hurry. He became extremely panicked, thinking, "Why am I here?" His memory had failed him because now he was truly lost. He looked into the next few rooms hoping to find a nurse or a doctor to help him. His panic kept growing, and he was starting to feel a tightening in his chest.

In her hospital bed, Betty was wondering where Julian was. Knowing that his memory was not as sharp as it had been even six months earlier, she started to worry. She asked her doctor to look for him since he might be lost. Before her heart surgery, she could still take care of him in their home, but now she worried if she would be too weak. To make things worse, Julian had started to depend on her more and more, even for minor things.

Her doctor was at the nurse's station to ask the nurses if anyone had seen Julian just as he was struggling down the hall.

"Mr. Fairless, Betty is in room 504," the doctor said as he grasped Julian's hand and led him a couple of rooms down the hall. When Julian saw his wife, he was shaking and instantly ran over and hugged her! But his panic had overtaken his body, and he died instantly in her arms of a massive heart attack.

He was fortunate. His Alzheimer's disease had only become noticeable several years earlier. In hindsight, the signs of the disease had been observed by family members about six years before his death.

Why do I think my grandfather was fortunate? I watched my Grandmother Sylvia's downward progression with the disease over a fifteen-year period of time. For the last five years of her life, my grandmother, as we knew her, was gone. Those last five years were excruciating for my family, especially for my uncles who were her caregivers. She had anger issues, could not recognize anyone, and experienced hallucinations. Those were only some of the problems she exhibited. The five years before that time were heartbreaking as the disease slowly took over her mind; sometimes she was herself, but other times she would become confused and angry. She would often wake up in the middle of the night, and either she did not know where she was, or she could not find something and would frantically search for that missing item.

The first five years of her Alzheimer's disease were truly frustrating, as she wanted to keep her independence. She loved living alone and having the freedom to use her car, but she was gradually becoming a hazard to herself and others. One night, her neighbors found her running down the street frantically calling for her mother who had died almost thirty years before. Grandmother Sylvia routinely called 911 because she thought that people were either breaking into her home or that people were there who refused to leave. Invariably, when the police arrived there was no one to be found. After about five of these emergency calls, the police advised my uncles that she needed to be placed into someone's care because they could no longer respond to her calls. My uncles chose to take her into their home where they experienced her downward decline firsthand. Those of you with family members who have this disease are familiar with the heartrending progression of Alzheimer's disease.

My family is very worried about getting Alzheimer's disease—especially my mother and her brother, since both of their parents had the disease—and many Americans are worried as well. An Alzheimer's survey taken in 2010 for the MetLife Foundation revealed that Americans fear getting Alzheimer's disease almost as much as cancer, which is currently the most feared disease. More than half of those surveyed knew little or nothing about the disease. Since AD is predicted to mushroom with the advent of the aging baby boomers, knowledge of the disease, as well as tools to reduce the risk, will be beneficial for all of us.

1
~

Alzheimer's Disease (AD)

When the German neurologist Alois Alzheimer first identified Alzheimer's disease as a disorder in 1906, it was considered to be psychological, and the patient was most likely
institutionalized after the diagnosis. Nowadays, it is known to
be a degenerative neurological disease characterized by a particular set of changes in the brain that, once started, are pro-
gressive and irreversible.

Dementia and Alzheimer's

Dementia is not a disease in itself but rather a term used to
describe a group of symptoms. These symptoms may include
the decline of mental functions such as memory, reasoning,
and language ability, as well as changes in personality, mood,
and behavior. Dementia develops when parts of the brain are
injured or diseased. There are over fifty known causes of dementia, and most of them are quite rare.

Alzheimer's disease (AD) is the most common cause of dementia. Other major causes of dementia from degenerative
neurological diseases are Parkinson's disease, Huntington's
disease, and some types of multiple sclerosis. Vascular demen-

1

tia can be caused by multiple strokes in the brain. Traumatic head injuries caused by motor vehicle accidents, falls, or numerous hits to the brain as seen in football players and boxers can cause dementia. Dementia may also be caused by infections of the central nervous system such as meningitis and HIV. Even nutritional deficiencies, depression, the chronic use of alcohol, or drug abuse can cause dementia. Alzheimer's disease represents over half of all causes of dementia. Alzheimer's disease is an extremely complicated and devastating disease. It is complicated in that it involves related yet separate parts of the brain that combine to manifest the disease. Understanding how these separate parts of the brain become dysfunctional enough to produce a cascading effect that corrodes the brain is very complicated indeed. This corrosion leads at first to cell dysfunction, then to a loss of areas of the brain that communicate within itself, and eventually to a loss of communication between the brain and the entire body. As many of us have witnessed, the result is a human being who has lost all of his or her dependability and proficiency.

Research has shown that the road to memory loss in our senior years may start as early as our teen years! All of us begin our lives with clear arteries, but before some of us finish our adolescence, fatty streaks (cholesterol and other lipids that have accumulated on the arterial walls) have already begun to appear. By early adulthood these fatty streaks turn into fibrous plaques that begin to calcify and become raised lesions (Berenson, G., et al., 1998). As we age, these lesions may become sites of low-grade, chronic inflammation. The lesions eventually grow larger and more numerous, restricting blood flow throughout the body. Blood restriction is the hallmark of atherosclerosis, which is the leading cause of heart disease. Research suggests that the risk factors for heart disease such as diabetes, high blood pressure, a high-fat diet, elevated homocysteine levels, cigarette smoking, and a sedentary lifestyle are also factors in the development of AD (Snowdon, D., et al., 2000 and Weir and Molloy, 2000). Thus the evidence of plaque buildup, or atherosclerosis, in the teenaged years leads many researchers to speculate that AD plaque may start its gradual corrosive process that early, as well. Nutritionally, this finding indicates that a diet that is good for the heart is also good for the brain.

How is Alzheimer's Disease Identified?

Let's look at the major players of this complex brain game in order to appreciate the complicated interaction of the players that slowly overwhelm the mental and physical aspects of our being once AD has taken over. The main players are β-amyloid plaques, neurofibrillary tangles, oxidative stress, and chronic inflammation. The β-amyloid plaques are widely perceived to be the start of the problem. They are derived from the amyloid precursor protein (APP). It is a simple protein that is found in the lipid membrane that surrounds all cells. APP activities are regulated by cholesterol found in these lipid membranes (Cordy, Hooper, and Turner, 2006). Under normal cellular conditions an enzyme called α-secretase cuts the APP first, and then another enzyme γ-secretase cuts it into a soluble protein of forty amino acids (the building blocks of proteins) in length. This soluble protein called α-amyloid is harmlessly secreted from the lipid membrane into the extracellular space to perform its role in cell growth, cell-to-cell communication, and as a contributor to cellular repair (Whitbourne, S., 2002). Our dynamic metabolism is continually responding to changes and therefore the APP, with its wide range of activities, has developed an alternate enzyme to cut it. In the alternative pathway, APP is first cut by β-secretase and then by γ-secretase. This action produces a soluble protein fragment that is approximately forty-two amino acids long, called β-amyloid (Aβ). But when Aβ combines with other Aβ proteins, it becomes insoluble and sticky.

The two different pathways for APP are:
APP→α-secretase→γ-secretase→α-amyloid (~40 amino acids)
APP→β-secretase→γ-secretase→β-amyloid (~42 amino acids)

Both of these proteins are normal derivatives of APP metabolism with roughly 90 percent of them being α-amyloid and 10 percent being Aβ. What role the Aβ type has is speculative at this time. It has been hypothesized that when they are still soluble, Aβ regulates brain cell growth similar to α-amyloid, but Aβ is associated with the growth at sites of injury or disease. These researchers hypothesize that as we age, factors like heart disease, diabetes, injury, a sedentary lifestyle, or most likely a combination of effects that cause the brain's metabolism to decline, produce an increase in Aβ to facilitate brain cell growth at damaged areas (Struble, R., et al., 2010).

It is also known that Aβ plaques become poisonous or toxic when they combine together or aggregate, and this combination can damage the nerve cells. This toxic aggregation might occur to signal the immune system to clear the used Aβ from the extracellular space through the activation of the macrophages and, exclusive to the brain, microglia. Both the macrophages and the microglia are considered to be the janitors of the immune system. Unfortunately, as we age these janitors may become faulty and may not adequately remove the cells' waste products (Fiala, M., et al, 2005). Therefore, as the many risk factors of aging start accumulating and the brain's metabolism declines, the percentage of toxic, insoluble Aβ peptides increases. As these insoluble Aβ aggregates add up, they slowly become compact spherical structures in the brain called senile plaques. A wide range of research is ongoing to stop APP from ever engaging in the alternate β/γ–secretase pathway (Vassar, R., et al., 2009). But if the above hypothesis is correct, increasing the brain's metabolic activity should be the goal. Prevention and nutrition become important in order to keep our immune system healthy and our brain's metabolism active.

While these senile plaques are building up outside the brain cells (called neurons), inside the cells, even more devastating action is occurring. Insoluble neurofibrillary tangles (NFT) are forming, most likely caused by repeated internal and external neuron damage. The damage occurs by a process known as oxidative stress, slowly killing the neuron by disrupting its basic mechanisms. Where do these abnormal tangles come from? The neuronal cell structure is called the cytoskeletal system (cyto means cell), and it is made up of filaments and microtubules. These filaments and microtubules have other proteins associated with them that cross–link with them for support. Think of the filaments and microtubules as the steel beams of a large building, with the floors being the cross–linking proteins.

One of these cross–linking proteins is a prime suspect in AD. Its name is tau, and it belongs to a family of proteins appropriately called microtubule associated proteins (MAP). This whole MAP family of proteins is found throughout the body and brain as structural components of cells, including the tau protein. In a normal neuron, tau's role is to bind and support the microtubule assembly in the long branches of the neurons called axons, and to a lesser degree in the neuron's central body. The tau protein's role is extremely important because it supports the neuron's structure, which allows intracellular communication and the transport of nutrients throughout the neuron and its numerous long axons.

Unfortunately, tau may undergo dangerous biochemical modifications that result in what is called hyperphosphorylation, a change that makes tau nonfunctional. This change causes, among other things, the loss of the whole filament/microtubule assembly. All these filaments and microtubules then stick together—having lost their support—and form the insoluble NFTs. Ultimately, the whole cytoskeletal system breaks down, killing the cell. These biochemical modifications are also believed to be caused by a decrease in metabolic activity that leads to oxidative stress, which is the third member of the AD team.

The Role of Oxidative Stress

The natural mechanism of the immune system is activated when a cell is in distress or when foreign invaders are detected. This activation may be beneficial to the cell because either the distress is brought under control and any damage is repaired, or the foreign invaders are captured and eliminated. If the damage is too great, however, the immune system goes into overdrive trying to salvage the cell or group of cells. The term "positive feedback loop" means that over the years, depending on the damage or "oxidative stress," the immune system grows out of control as it tries to repair the cells. This effort produces even more damage, which causes the immune system to send in more immune molecules, and the cycle repeats over and over again. Numerous hypotheses regard chronic oxidative stress suffered over a lifetime to be a contributing factor in Alzheimer's disease (Sultana, Perluigi, and Butterfield, 2006).

What is oxidation and oxidative stress? An oxidant is a molecule that accepts, or in the case of "free radicals," steals an electron from another molecule. Oxygen is an oxidant that we see in action all the time. When an apple slice turns brown or butter turns rancid, it is because oxygen has interacted with their cells. When copper gets that green patina or metal turns to rust, you can thank oxygen for those changes. Oxygen is nature's way of breaking things down so that they can decompose—as in the case of rotting fruit. Yet oxygen is vital to the body and brain. The oxygen that we inhale goes from our lungs to the blood stream where it combines with glucose (or other fuels) to produce energy for the whole body, and especially the brain. Most of the time, oxygen metabolizes very efficiently within each of our cells, resulting in a balanced exchange of electrons. These interactions are termed "oxidation" (accepting electrons) and "reduction" (the loss of electrons). The interactions actually happen simultaneously and are a natural process that is necessary to keep the body healthy.

Free Radicals

Conversely, a very small percentage of oxygen interactions may create an unstable reactive molecule. That instability occurs when a molecule is left with an unpaired electron—known as a "free radical"—during the electron exchange with oxygen. These unstable free radicals steal electrons from the body's healthy molecules in order to balance their electrons and stabilize themselves. These interactions are also called oxidation, but this kind of oxidation is not a balanced, simultaneous exchange of electrons that creates a stable molecule. Instead, the unstable free radical may start a chain reaction, because the molecule from which it stole the electron becomes a new free radical. That new free radical steals an electron from another molecule, and so the chain reaction proceeds. Unfortunately, during the time the molecules are free radicals searching for an electron with which to pair, they cause a great deal of damage to different parts of one or many cells.

Especially hard hit are the cell's lipid membranes. This damage is dangerous because the cell's membrane is its barrier to the extracellular environment. If the oxidation happens inside the cell, its DNA, RNA, lipids, and proteins may also be damaged, having enormous implications for the everyday functioning of the cell. The body does have a defense against these free radicals, and they are antioxidants. Antioxidants give the free radicals the electrons they need in order to stop the radical oxidants from causing more damage and generating more free radicals. "Oxidative stress" is defined as the unbalance between free radical oxidants and antioxidants, *favoring* the oxidant to the point that exceeds the body's ability to defend itself against such damage. Oxidative stress promotes a host of chronic diseases. Nutrition has a major role to play in oxidative stress, as well.

Oxidants and Antioxidants

A healthy immune system keeps up with normal, reactive oxygen species interactions. It also handles the variety of other reactions that generate free radicals formed normally in cells as they continuously use carbohydrates, fats, and proteins for energy and other normal metabolic functions. Oxygen is not the only molecule that causes oxidation; a number of other factors contribute to the generation of free radicals that come from external sources. The major contributors are environmental contaminants, our modern diet, and the stress of our lifestyles. These external sources may overwhelm the body's natural antioxidant defense system leading to oxidative stress. Even our healthy immune system generates free radicals to combat what it perceives as foreign invaders.

One of many tools the immune system uses is a tactic called "oxidative burst" produced by specialized cells called phagocytes. To kill a bacteria or virus, a phagocyte blasts the invader with many free radicals—called hydroxyl radicals—that are derived from hydrogen peroxide. This blast kills the invader and also sends out hydroxyl radicals that miss the invader. The hydroxyl radicals continue to actively search for an electron with which to pair. These free radicals have the potential to damage healthy cells and tissues if not stopped right away. Fortunately, a healthy immune system can handle these attacks. When we have a cold or flu virus, the symptoms we experience are the result of the immune system fighting back and repairing the damage so that the body can recover.

The brain, however, is different from the rest of the body in that it is highly vulnerable to oxidative damage. This difference is due to the brain's immense energy needs. The brain has a high oxygen consumption as well as a high lipid content and retains relatively few natural antioxidants compared to other organs in the body. Unless ample supplies of antioxidants are continually made available through our diet, the external sources of free radicals can easily overwhelm the brain's defense system, causing unwanted oxidative stress.

In the twenty-first century, we need to consume more antioxidants than we did a hundred years ago because of the many toxic free radical generators that we encounter each day. Cigarette smoke and air pollution are huge free radical generators; pesticides, additives, and preservatives in our food and water supplies also harbor many sources of free radicals. And now we are learning that hazardous chemicals used in the production of food products do not have to be recorded on the ingredient list because they are considered to be "components in a production procedure" by the US Department of Agriculture (USDA). Prime examples are the ammonia in "pink slime" beef and arsenic in fruit juices. It has also been revealed that hazardous chemicals employed in the manufacturing of products that we use are everywhere in our environment—even inside our tissues and cells. Examples are the chemicals bisphenol A (BPA) found in plastics and in the lining of food containers and fire retardants used in clothing, curtains, and upholstered furniture. Cumulative oxidative damage in the brain over a lengthy period of time might activate pathways that lead to cell death (called apoptosis). This process may cause the brain to shrink, which leads to dementia. If oxidative damage does begin in one's twenties, this factor might account for the slow progression of the disease and the later life onset of AD that is not related to genetic factors.

Inflammation—Friend and Foe

The last major player in Alzheimer's disease is the captain of the team: inflammation. Inflammation is an active part of the immune system where the response may vary greatly, depending on the playing field. This team captain is playing to win at any cost because every cell in the whole body depends on the captain for protection. Inflammation is the body's best defense against an enemy, whether it is an injury, an infection, or an invading pathogen. Antioxidants cruising throughout the body are the first line of this defense. They give up their electrons to stop free radicals as part of their job, with new recruits taking over as the used up ones retire. When the system is overwhelmed due to oxidative stress and there are no new antioxidant recruits, damage to the cells occurs. A distress signal is sent out to the immune system. Localized tissue hormones called prostaglandins, which are important to the whole immune system, send out the distress signals. While the remaining antioxidants are working hard to minimize the damage, inflammation is preparing its team by calling on the immune response to examine the damage, help isolate the area, and mobilize immune molecules to the site of the damage. Pro-inflammatory genes are also activated, leading to the release of immune molecules called cytokines, chemokines, and adhesion molecules. Counter regulatory or anti-inflammatory pathways are simultaneously activated to keep the inflammatory response under control. This activation allows repair and healing to take place after the attack. When the inflammatory response is acute, the inflammation will last only a few days, similar to getting a cut or contracting the flu. But low-grade, chronic inflammation may last for several weeks, months, or even years. Chronic inflammation renders the counter anti-inflammatory pathways inadequate in order to control the immune system's response, and repair is never fully completed because of the positive feedback loop. This chronic inflammation may lead to excessive damage to cell membranes, proteins, lipids, DNA, and RNA. The damage may be so severe that it compromises tissue and organ functions as in the cases of arteriosclerosis, arthritis, tumor development, and dementia.

The Amazing Body

To summarize the predicament: oxidation that generates a free radical under normal cell metabolism is controlled naturally by antioxidants and a healthy immune system. External causes of oxidation that have increased over the last hundred years of civilization have taxed the natural antioxidants to the point where oxidative stress has occurred more frequently, damaging neurons in the process. The immune response is activated, inflammation is initiated to repair the injury, and the Aβ protein is increased to assist the damaged neurons to generate new growth. As we age and the AD risk factors causing the immune system and brain metabolism to decline increase, the Aβ peptides are not adequately cleared from the brain and thus cause toxic aggregates. This process causes more damage, more inflammation, and an endless destructive cycle of damage and partial repair. That cycle, among other problems, causes tau to become inoperable, and the cytoskeleton falls apart, resulting in the death of neurons.

Do not despair or believe that there is nothing anyone can do about the damage that might have started in our twenties. The body is amazing. When given the correct tools, it can repair itself and function optimally in a relatively short amount of time. Edgar Cayce's readings indicated that every cell in the body will have been rebuilt over a seven-year period, so you will have a new body every seven years. You have the choice for health or disease every day. There are simple lifestyle changes you can make immediately so that in as little as six months, you may be able to redirect your body and importantly, your brain, toward better health. After seven years, your body will have rebuilt each one of its cells according to all of your healthful changes, and you will be functioning at your best and brightest!

2

~

The Problem

Alzheimer's disease (AD) is on the rise not only in the United States, where over 5.4 million Americans have experienced the disease as of 2011, but also worldwide. The World Health Organization warned that AD might affect sixteen million Americans and possibly 115 million people worldwide by 2050. According to the National Institute of Aging in the United States, one in eight baby boomers will experience AD in their later years of life. The countless numbers of people who will develop AD represent a crisis. Additionally, because of the long duration of the disease and the high cost of managing it, AD poses one of the greatest challenges to our society medically, economically, and emotionally. Prevention may be the best tool to defend against this frightening disease.

Why the Increase?

What is contributing to this accelerating rate of incidences of AD? Interestingly enough, the major contributing factor is that we are living longer and healthier lives. Age is the foremost risk factor for Alzheimer's disease that is not related to genetic factors; people over the age of eighty-five have a 30 percent chance of showing signs of dementia. Our great-grandparents typically died of complications from heart disease or cancer in their sixties or seventies, and therefore the incidence of AD was low. To date, there is no evidence that AD is spreading throughout the baby boomer population other than the fact that Americans are living longer. Simply put, there are now more middle-aged people at risk for brain aging conditions once they reach their eighties or nineties. At present, the average life expectancy is eighty-seven years and is expected to climb steadily. Living over a century is no longer rare. Longevity has come about through better health care and pharmaceuticals, a larger variety of food choices, readily available supplements for every health concern, an increased awareness of the importance of exercise, and the reduction of cigarette smoking. On a side note, current smokers are 50 percent *more* likely to develop AD or other dementias then those who do not smoke or those who are past smokers (Reitz, C., et al., 2007). Even though old age is the number one risk factor, there is another side to the increase of Alzheimer's disease. Mental disorders like dementia do not represent the process of normal aging. Memory loss is normal in older people but that does not mean that they have dementia. Today many people age gracefully into their nineties and beyond without any signs of AD or other dementia. There must be other environmental and lifestyle reasons for the enormous predicted increase of this devastating disease.

Over the last one hundred years or so, our world has become more and more industrialized, most of which has been to our benefit; but unknown health consequences have arisen that are now highlighted because of our long lives. Beneficial advances have been made in animal husbandry, synthetic fertilizer and pesticide use, and most importantly, in food processing and distribution. Instead of raising our own animals or produce, which is hard work and time consuming, everything has become readily available at the local grocery store. One disadvantage is that consumers have thousands of overly processed and refined food choices. Another disadvantage includes the fact that modern animal husbandry has changed the composition of the fat content of farm animals. These animals were taken from the field where they grazed on grass to be raised in warehouses were they consume corn and soybean products while receiving antibiotics and growth hormones. Synthetic fertilizers and pesticides have made their way into our tissues, a problem we are not equipped to handle because our bodies can not break them down so these chemicals can then build up inside our cells and disrupt their activities. Processed and refined foods have lost their natural nutritional composition because most of their nutrients have been stripped away or destroyed. Consuming these foods leads to poor assimilation of whatever nutrients are left after processing. Though some vital nutrients are added back into foods after processing, these nutrients are usually synthetic and are poorly assimilated, if at all. Distribution often leaves even wholesome foods such as fruits and vegetables with little or no nutrient content because the minute these foods are harvested, they start to lose their nutritive benefits—especially the vitamins. If foods travel long distances and then wait in a warehouse before going to a store, most of the nutrients have decayed by the time they get to our homes (Jensen and Anderson, 1990).

There is also the problem of convenience. It is much easier, and sometimes more economical, to throw something into the microwave oven or to obtain meals from a fast-food restaurant—especially a drive-through establishment—when life gets too busy for cooking at home. Shopping, preparing, and cooking food takes time, and time is a luxury some households think they cannot afford. Some people believe it is too much trouble to cook all of the time—or at all—and are unaware that their choice of convenient foods is unhealthy, while others have no idea how to cook, opting for prepackaged foods rather than starvation. There are also those people who live in what are called the "food deserts" of inner cities, where food choices are limited because there are no local grocery stores. Instead, there are many fast-food restaurants and convenience stores that usually do not carry fresh foods. Even more disturbing is that over the last two decades, fast foods and sugary drinks have become a dominant part of the food culture at an ever-earlier age. This trend has created an unbalanced chemical makeup in many people, with the unknown health consequences resulting in a host of chronic diseases. The main examples are heart disease, strokes, obesity, type 2 diabetes, many types of cancer, Alzheimer's disease, and other dementias.

Biochemistry out of Balance

One example of an unbalanced chemical is glucose. Glucose is a simple sugar or simple carbohydrate found in abundance in our modern food supply and might be one of the culprits responsible for the decline of cognitive function. Glucose is vital to the brain because it is the brain's preferred energy source. For instance, the energy that glucose provides is required for the synthesis, release, and uptake of neurotransmitters such as serotonin, norepinephrine, and acetylcholine (a neurotransmitter that is known to be low in AD patients). As a result of this unbalance, metabolic conditions may interfere with the brain's ability to obtain and utilize glucose. Although the brain will try to adapt through the use of other fuels, low glucose levels cause a decline in the brain's overall metabolic activity.

What "metabolic conditions" interfere with glucose's availability to the brain if it is so abundant in today's foods? This abundance is the problem—there is too much of a good thing! You might notice that if you read the nutritional facts of foods, glucose is not listed. Nevertheless, it is there—hidden in ingredients like sugar, brown sugar, sucrose, dextrose, maltose, corn syrup, and high fructose corn sugar.

Carbohydrates

Let's have a short lesson on carbohydrates to understand the importance of glucose. Dietary carbohydrates are either simple carbohydrates (sugars) or complex carbohydrates (starches and fibers). The building blocks of all carbohydrates are three sugars: glucose, fructose, and galactose. Fructose is the sweetest of the sugars and is found naturally in fruit and honey. Galactose binds together with glucose to form lactose, or milk sugar. Fructose and galactose will be converted to glucose in the liver. Glucose is the most abundant sugar in nature, and it is found in all plants as starch. Starch is the way that plants store their glucose for energy, which is in long chains of hundreds or thousands of glucose molecules. Since all animals consume some plants, glucose is the main energy source for almost every living thing. When a body consumes plants, the complex carbohydrates (starch and fiber, along with their associated minerals and vitamins) are slowly digested, and the glucose is released at a modest, regulated rate so that the blood glucose levels rise only slightly. Starches like those found in white flour, white rice, and all the other processed and refined starch products behave more like simple carbohydrates because their long chains of glucose have been broken down and stripped of their fiber and nutrients. As a result, they digest quickly, causing a surge in blood glucose levels. When you consume a meal, all of these simple and complex carbohydrates will be broken down so that the glucose can be used for energy immediately—anywhere in the body—or stored in the liver and muscles, ready to release their supplies when blood glucose levels drop between meals or during physical exercise or work. Any excess glucose goes into longer-term storage. This storage happens after a few modifications are made to glucose to become fat and then placed into fat (adipose) cells for future energy needs.

The Link between Diabetes and AD

Diabetes is the major metabolic condition involving glucose, with the hormone insulin being at the core of the problem. Excessive glucose consumption along with a diet high in protein can lead to type 2 diabetes. Why? Protein and carbohydrates regulate each other. This balance is maintained when consuming a meal of plant proteins and complex carbohydrates—for example, brown rice and beans. The balance becomes lopsided when consuming too much meat, a highly concentrated protein, which causes a sugar craving as the metabolism attempts to reestablish its protein/carbohydrate balance. Additionally, consuming a great deal of glucose increases the desire for more protein to retain the balance; and as this cycle continues, overeating and obesity may occur. Maintaining this balance when there is too much glucose in the system may cause the pancreas to produce a large amount of the hormone insulin, which regulates glucose. The overproduction of insulin causes the body cells and the brain neurons to become less sensitive or resistant to the insulin, triggering glucose levels to rise even more. This rise in glucose levels stimulates the pancreatic cells to make even more insulin, eventually exhausting the pancreas and its ability to function at all. Obesity and insulin resistance have recently been associated with cognitive decline and

Alzheimer's disease. The growing prevalence of obesity today, especially among younger people where it is estimated that one third of the population is obese, raises the possibility that AD and other dementias may activate at earlier ages (Hildreth, Van Pelt, and Schwartz, 2012).

One characterization of Alzheimer's disease is a *decrease* in glucose metabolism and brain metabolic activity in some areas of the brain due to inadequate levels of glucose. These areas also have numerous neurofibrillary tangles. This feature suggests that an altered energy balance may induce tau to become abnormal, which makes the neuronal cytoskeletal system more prone to oxidation. Consequently, the death cycle begins because the cell is starving from a lack of glucose (Planel, E., et al., 2001).

Cortisol—Another Friend and Foe

Cortisol, the so-called "stress hormone" since it is involved with the "fight-or-flight" response, is another chemical that may become unbalanced, causing a metabolic condition. Cortisol also regulates glucose. Too much glucose means the body has to generate a great deal of cortisol to control the glucose. Couple this work to control glucose with a stressful lifestyle that is constantly generating cortisol because of the fight-or-flight response, and a biochemical disaster is in the making. This increase in cortisol has negative effects on many systems; in particular, it increases blood pressure and blocks important inflammation messengers that disrupt the immune system. The reason for the increased blood pressure is that cortisol puts the body on high alert so that it is ready to fight or flee in response to what it perceives as a threat. This response means that the body needs more energy, which is why cortisol helps to regulate glucose. Cortisol not only shuts down the immune system but also impairs the digestive system. Both of these systems use a great deal of energy that the body might need in order to fight or run (take flight) from a threat. Cortisol is a necessary hormone during times of physical danger such as our ancestors might have experienced when confronted by an angry bear or a ravenous lion. Unfortunately, it is also activated whenever we experience any stress, ranging in degree from being late to an appointment to worrying about a loved one who must go off to war.

Limit Your Advanced Glycation End Products (AGEs)

In diabetes, or whenever refined sugar is consumed, another meta-bolic condition may occur, which is the glycation of proteins (Munch, Deuther–Conrad, and Gasic–Milenkovic, 2002). Glycation happens when blood sugar levels are too high, triggering glucose to bind to a protein. Glycation generates abnormal proteins that may do enormous damage when incorporated into cell and tissues. During the glycation process, free radicals are generated, known as "advanced glycation end products" (AGEs). These AGEs are a possible source of oxidative stress. This type of oxidative stress occurs particularly in people with a diet high in refined sugars and starches or, in the case of diabetes, in people with insulin resistance and/or pancreas malfunction. The glycation of proteins and their free radical AGEs have an external source, as well. Whenever meats are subjected to high heat, such as being grilled, fried, or overcooked, glycation and AGEs are generated. The high heat oxi-dizes the proteins, and then they bind with the glucose in the meat. When these foods are consumed, most of the abnormal proteins are not utilized and are discarded before they are digested, but the AGEs are still there, increasing the body's oxidative stress. And as previously stated, oxidative stress is considered to be a causative factor in AD.

The Fat Problem

Another health issue that has become identified in the last twenty years is the potential harm to our bodies produced by some of the fats and oils in our diets. We now realize that not all fats are created equal: some fats are "bad" and some fats are not only "good" but also neces-sary and even essential for our health and well-being. This knowledge was unrecognized until recently when scientists started researching fats during the 1970s. The problem began during the industrial age when it became easier to obtain butter and lard around the turn of the century. Several decades later, health officials began to correlate high levels of cholesterol in the blood with the occurrence of heart disease. In the 1950s, a campaign was launched to direct the American diet away from butter and lard toward other fats that were supposed to be healthier (like margarine and other inexpensive vegetable oils that did not contain cholesterol). One of the most unfortunate shifts was the recommended use of margarine. Margarine was produced with hydrogenated vegetable oils to make it solid so that it behaved like butter or lard. This shift in fats resulted in a whole host of biochemical problems that will be discussed in chapter three.

A Whole Food Revolution

Some people started to notice these problems in the 1980s, and they wanted an alternative. These individuals started demanding organic fruits, whole grains and vegetables, organic cold, expeller-pressed vegetable oil, organic free-range fowl, and pasture-fed meat and dairy products. This trend prompted the term "whole foods" to become used in the 1990s. Along with this movement, people wanted to "buy local" so that the foods they bought did not have to be shipped from faraway places and would therefore retain most of their nutrients. There was also the desire to lessen the environmental impact of these shipped products. Farmers' markets have sprung up all around the country, allowing people to purchase fresh and locally grown foods as well as products like honey or cut flowers. At present, there are many opportunities to enjoy organic products in restaurants and from mail order sources or specialty grocery stores, and most regular grocery stores carry some organic produce along with other organic products. The next phase of this movement will be to serve children healthier meals at school, to lower the cost of organic products so that they become a better choice than less expensive but overly processed products, and to encourage people to start gardening in order to grow their own nutritious, whole foods. Another excellent idea is the neighborhood garden party where neighbors exchange their gardens' overabundance with each other and then share a meal where everyone contributes a specialty item made from the garden or farm. Many food banks currently accept items grown in local gardens, helping the gardener who has an overabundance of fruits and vegetables as well as the food bank's recipients who welcome more fresh foods.

The whole food revolution has helped to change our attitude towards food by making us realize that we are what we eat and that our very health depends on the quality of our food. This realization has been lost in the world of commercialized food production. Whole foods are slowly making a comeback, along with an emphasis on the importance of our health and well-being. As Edgar Cayce stated, "... what we think and what we eat—combined together—*make* what we *are*; physically and mentally." (288-38)

3
~

The Nuts and the Oil of It

What you consume today, no matter how young you are, may ultimately determine your risk for Alzheimer's disease (AD) in your senior years. Current research now considers type 2 diabetes and heart disease to be known risk factors for AD. Both of these conditions may be caused by an improper diet and controlled by adopting a nutritious diet. New studies are also offering evidence that dietary choices might possibly prevent mental decline or at least slow its progress.

The Mediterranean Diet

One of these choices is the Mediterranean diet (Scarmeas, N., et al., 2009). Most of us have heard that the Mediterranean diet is one of the best diet models to follow to prevent the development of type 2 diabetes and heart disease. One imagines the Mediterranean diet to be comprised of abundant fresh vegetables (especially tomatoes), plenty of pasta, and lots of olive oil—and it is! At present, there is considerable evidence that walnuts and fish may actually be the keys to this healthful diet (Galli and Marangoni, 2006). What do walnuts and fish have in common? Both have an abundance of a "good" fat called omega-3.

The Good-For-You Fats

Omega-3 is a polyunsaturated fatty acid that is essential to our diet because the body does not make it. We must obtain omega-3 fatty acids from the foods we consume. Most importantly, this is one fat you should not avoid since it never goes into making body fat; only saturated fats and trans fats do that! Instead, omega-3 fats are used to make many biologically active compounds that affect the entire body, such as those that regulate blood pressure and the immune system.

Omega-3 fats are especially important in brain functioning because they are involved with the production of neurotransmitters. The membranes of every cell in our bodies contain omega-3 fats, with brain cells having the highest amount. In fact, two thirds of the entire brain is composed of fatty acids, with omega-3 being the most prevalent. Another important function of omega-3 is to keep blood vessels fit and flexible. Having healthy blood vessels means that we are less likely to develop hardening of the arteries. Hardening of the arteries is a major contributor to heart disease and therefore to Alzheimer's disease, as well.

Sources of Omega-3 Fats

The best sources of omega-3s for a healthful diet are fatty fish such as salmon, cod, tuna, herring, halibut, trout, sardines, anchovies, eel, and even caviar. Beware of farm-raised fish; they have virtually no omega-3 fats because the fish are not raised on a natural fish diet. Shellfish like shrimp, crab, and lobster are also low in omega-3 fats because they are almost fat-free naturally. The best non-fish sources of omega-3 fats are freshly ground flaxseeds and flaxseed oil. Other foods high in omega-3 fats are pumpkin seeds, wheat germ, walnuts, and the oils from all of these, as well as canola oil. There are other good sources that are not widely known because they are not considered high-fat foods. The little fat they do have is high in omega-3s, and these include broccoli, cantaloupe, cauliflower, chard, Chinese cabbage, grape leaves, kale, kidney beans, parsley, spinach, and wheat-grass.

Eggs Are Back in Favor

The hottest new item that is full of omega-3 fats is the *egg*! Don't choose just any egg, which is high in saturated fats since the chickens in commercial operations are fed a corn-based diet (corn contains no omega-3 fats); instead, eat organic eggs from cage-free, vegetarian fed chickens raised with a diet high in omega-3 fats. There are also eggs available in grocery stores that are high in DHA (a type of omega-3 fat that is good for your brain) because the chickens' food has been enriched with it. All these organic eggs contain omega-3 fats and 25 percent less saturated fat than regular eggs and another important benefit is that these chickens do not need antibiotics or added hormones.

Organic, free-range chickens, turkey, and ducks that eat their natural diets are very healthful to consume, too. This is also true for cattle, pigs, and lambs. If fed their natural grass diets, which are loaded with omega-3 fats along with vitamins, minerals, and antioxidants, the animals do not need antibiotics or hormones because their bodies naturally take care of themselves! Another important benefit with the new omega-3 egg versus the regular egg is that it is higher in lutein, vitamin E, and folate, and as an added bonus, they contain vitamin B-6, vitamin B-12, iodine, and zinc. Along with its complete protein composition, superior taste, and only seventy calories, the organic egg is truly an exceptional food choice!

The Truth About Cholesterol

You might have noticed that I have not mentioned the cholesterol content of eggs, which is the reason they fell out of favor. Let's have a quick cholesterol lesson. We are familiar with the two types of cholesterol *vehicles* (there is only one *kind* of cholesterol) that are important for health: the low-density lipoproteins (LDLs) and the high-density lipoproteins (HDLs). Since oil and water do not mix, the proteins surround the various fats or lipids so that they can be circulated in the watery bloodstream. Both LDLs and HDLs transport mainly cholesterol but also other lipids; and in the case of LDLs, the fat-soluble vitamins A and E are transported, as well. LDLs circulate throughout the body and brain to deliver their contents so that the cells can build new membranes, replenish their vitamin A and E stocks, and make hormones and other compounds as needed. The problem with LDLs—and why they are considered "bad"—is that as they travel through the blood, their cholesterol is vulnerable to attack by free radicals. If the blood stream has an abundance of antioxidants, the damage is minimal; but if there are inadequate amounts of antioxidants, the oxidized cholesterol may start forming the fatty streaks on the artery walls, leading to atherosclerosis. The "good" HDLs perform the opposite function; they circulate through the body and pick up the used cholesterol and other lipids from the cells, bringing them back to the liver for recycling or disposal. LDLs and HDLs are neither bad nor good; they are necessary blood-transport vehicles for cholesterol. LDLs and HDLs are not found in foods—only cholesterol itself is.

The truth is that it is *not* the cholesterol in whole foods that causes high blood cholesterol levels and atherosclerosis. The culprit is a diet high in saturated animal fat, refined carbohydrates, and processed foods containing oxidized cholesterol and a body with low levels of systemic antioxidants. Nevertheless, there are certain people who are genetically predisposed to high cholesterol levels who *should* avoid food sources of cholesterol. Your liver converts these saturated animal fats and fragments from carbohydrates and proteins into cholesterol at the high-end rate of 50,000,000,000,000,000 molecules per minute (Whitney and Rolfes, 2002). Therefore the amount of cholesterol from our diet is very small compared to what the liver produces.

Having a high LDL blood count is bad because your liver is being pressured into making a lot of cholesterol from an excess of saturated animal fats and sugar. A low HDL blood count is bad because there are not enough of the lipoproteins to take away the used cholesterol so your total blood cholesterol levels rise.

Consider eating a breakfast consisting only of two boiled eggs, or coddled eggs. Coddled is a special way to cook eggs that Edgar Cayce recommended because the cooking process pampers, or coddles, the eggs to preserve all the nutrients. To make coddled eggs, simply boil enough water that will cover the eggs, and then with a spoon gently lower the eggs, still shelled, into the pot. Now, turn off the heat to let the eggs rest for five to ten minutes, and then enjoy these nutritious eggs. Compare this breakfast of coddled eggs to a breakfast of fried eggs and bacon accompanied by either toast spread with butter (or worse, margarine) and jelly or by pancakes topped with butter and syrup. The first coddled egg breakfast will not raise your cholesterol levels, but the second breakfast undoubtedly will since all the ingredients required for generating more cholesterol are present: saturated animal fats, refined carbohydrates, and protein. You do not have to avoid bacon altogether, however. Edgar Cayce's readings indicated that very crisp bacon may be eaten guilt-free, on occasion, suggesting that once you cook all the saturated fat away from the actual meat, it is much better for the body. Cayce also mentioned other safe ways to prepare eggs besides coddling, including soft boiled, poached, or soft-scrambled—" . . . or prepared in any manner just so they are not fried in grease . . . " (306-3) The readings recommended against frying any food in grease, as well.

The Fat Difference

Even though it appears that the fat found in a particular animal or plant is one type of fat, an example would be the idea that beef is full of only saturated fats. Let's have a quick lesson in fat nomenclature. As noted before, fat is a general term for lipids. Fat is actually a subset of the lipid family, which includes the fatty acids (fats and oils) and phospholipids. The best known phospholipids are lecithin and sterols, one of which is cholesterol. Fatty acids are incorporated into triglycerides for use in the body. A triglyceride is comprised of three fatty acids attached to a glycerol molecule. Each of the three fatty acids may be either saturated or unsaturated. If there are more saturated fatty acids, the product is called a fat, such as butter. With more unsaturated fatty acids, the product becomes a liquid and is called an oil. Saturated fatty acids are straight chains of carbons with hydrogens attached with no double bonds. In other words, their carbons are saturated with hydrogen. Unsaturated fatty acids are also chains of carbons with hydrogens attached, but some of the carbons are missing hydrogen, creating double bonds between the carbons. The carbons are therefore not saturated with hydrogen—or unsaturated. Being unsaturated also makes them bend at these double bonds, which is important for their functions. It is a fact that only animals, even fish and shellfish, contain cholesterol, and that all plants do not contain cholesterol. Nevertheless, every animal and plant is a composition of saturated, monounsaturated, and polyunsaturated fats in a variety of combinations, depending on the food item. A good example is to compare the difference among feedlot beef (a four-ounce portion of prime rib), a four-ounce fillet of wild salmon, and a cup of raw broccoli.

Fat type	Saturated	Monounsaturated	Polyunsaturated	Cholesterol
Feedlot beef	16 grams	18 grams	1.5 grams	96 grams
Wild salmon	2.2 grams	0.6 grams	2.7 grams	98 grams
Broccoli	0.1 grams	0.5 grams	0.3 grams	0 grams

The living conditions in which a particular food is found also changes its fat composition. Examples are the aforementioned organic eggs, wild fish compared to farm-raised fish, or free-range animals compared to feedlot animals.

The Diet Difference

So what is in the Mediterranean diet that makes it so different from the typical American diet? The Mediterranean diet consists of a large amount of fruits, vegetables, beans, whole grains, nuts (mostly walnuts), and fish. Poultry, eggs, and dairy products are eaten in moderation. Red meat is rarely eaten, and it is usually pasture-fed lamb, which has considerably more omega-3 fats than feedlot animals. The main sources of fat originate from fish, nuts, and olive oil. One of many important studies found a favorable link between Alzheimer's disease and the Mediterranean diet. It demonstrated that people who closely followed the Mediterranean diet had a 40 percent to 60 percent lower risk of AD compared to those who did *not* follow the diet! (Scarmeas, N., et al., 2009).

How is this diet different from the typical American diet? In general, the difference is that the Mediterranean diet is high in fiber and low in saturated fats and processed foods, whereas the American diet is low in fiber and high in saturated fats and processed foods. Although the American diet is rapidly changing, most of us who were born before 1970 grew up eating what is called the "meat and potato" diet. The conventional wisdom at that time was that everyone should consume an animal protein at every meal or risk becoming malnourished, eventually withering away!

My mother, and her mother before her, adhered to the belief of eating meat and starches at every meal. I believe that my childhood family diet reflected this thinking for at least three generations. Breakfast consisted of eggs, bacon, or sausage and white bread toast with margarine and jelly or a sugary cereal with milk. Lunch usually consisted of a sandwich, also on white bread, made with mayonnaise or mustard, baloney, and processed American cheese. Dinner was the big meal of the day where the family ate together. Mom usually served some type of white bread and a salad first. We regularly had homemade biscuits that were so hard that my sister and I used to say they would kill anyone who was hit in the head with them! In order to soften up these biscuits, we put lots of margarine and jelly on them. The main course was typically beef or a meat dish consisting of hamburger, accompanied by potatoes or sometimes noodles, and a frozen or canned vegetable thrown in to complete the well-balanced meal. Sometimes, we had chicken or pork for a change, and luckily, fish on Fridays, although it was usually some type of fried fish. Turkey and fresh nuts were served only at Thanksgiving and Christmas, and we never had lamb. My mother's specialty was steak and potatoes—she must have known at the very least five different ways to cook those potatoes—and of course they had to be peeled! Baked potatoes were the only exception, but we were told not to eat the skin because it was grown in the ground, which would be like eating dirt! My mother did not know what Edgar Cayce knew, which is that most of the vitamins and minerals reside in the potato's skin. The starchy inside of the potato has very little nutrient content. Then, we make matters worse by piling them high with margarine and sour cream. To this day on Thanksgiving and Christmas, my mother begs me to peel the potatoes so that she doesn't have to pick out the peelings in front of the other guests!

The Bad Fats

This topic brings me to the last bit of unhealthy living that our generation's mothers unknowingly subjected us to—the use of cotton-seed oil, corn oil, and lard. Why are these oils a problem? The public was told around the time of the 1950s that products like margarine, Crisco (which is cottonseed oil, and before the invention of Crisco, humans had never consumed that kind of oil), and other low-cost vegetable oils including corn, sunflower, and soybean oils were healthier than butter. An intense campaign stated that the high cho-lesterol in butter was associated with heart disease and that the "solu-tion" was to begin using the "new products" that did not have any cholesterol. No one even considered using olive oil because everyone thought that olives belonged solely in martinis! The American popu-lation as a whole unquestionably adopted margarine as the spread of choice for breads, and everyone began to slather it on baked potatoes and other vegetables, as well. Crisco was used in baking those rich cakes, pies, and cookies that our mothers made from scratch. Corn or sunflower oil was used for frying foods such as chicken, potatoes, and tortillas. I shudder when I remember that my mother kept an old coffee can on the kitchen counter in which she saved the used bacon grease. At least she would dump it out and start fresh for another year during spring-cleaning! She actually added the grease into some dishes to make them "taste better," or she would use it on her baking pans to keep food from sticking. She would always use this bacon grease to fry chopped onions before adding them into the hamburger to cook for various dishes. I am sure she thought that a smidgen of this grease would do no harm, and I am also certain that she was not alone in this misguided idea.

Why wasn't the public informed that bacon grease was high in cho-lesterol? That secret was probably kept because lard was not available in grocery stores since it had fallen out of favor from bad press long before butter. The result was that people bought Crisco instead of lard and kept a can of bacon grease on their counters so that it would be ready to use at any moment! The danger of these oils was unknown at the time. Bacon grease slowly degrades and does not smell like rancid butter does, so no one recognized this used oil—cooked at high heat and then left out at room temperature for months—as being rancid. It was also not acknowledged that the cholesterol in the grease was oxidized and extremely toxic to blood vessels. Even before those years, Edgar Cayce's readings had recommended against the use of bacon grease for cooking.

Hydrogenation

At that time, no one knew that it was a major problem to hydrogenate oils to make products like margarine and Crisco behave like butter or to extend the shelf life of convenience foods. Hydrogenation was thought of as a "great solution" to the high cholesterol problem that Americans were facing. Food manufacturers took an inexpensive vegetable oil containing no cholesterol and made it not only solid like butter but also smoother and longer lasting at room temperature, all through the wonders of science! The scientists discovered long ago that this process creates two types of fats as hydrogen bubbles through the oil to harden it. One type of fat that is generated is configured as a normal fat, but the other type, known as a trans fat, becomes the opposite of normal, like a mirror image.

Trans Fats

These trans fats are not found in nature, much less in our bodies. Unfortunately, our cells have no choice but to utilize them if there is no better alternative fat source! Trans fats cause the cell membranes to misalign, leaving gaps that let in unwanted items like bacteria, viruses, and free radicals, and they also cause the membrane to be less flexible. A diet comprised of too many trans fats produced by hydrogenation contributes to unhealthy cells and overall to an unhealthy body. It is unfortunate that this "solution" to heart disease that was linked to high cholesterol has had such a harmful effect on our bodies. One of the outcomes is thought to be the sharp increase in inflammatory problems over the past thirty to fifty years. Some of these inflammatory conditions are arthritis, allergies, heart disease, stroke, and dementia. Most amazing is that the incidence of heart disease greatly increased with the use of these hydrogenated oils, which is the very problem that the "solution" was supposed to decrease!

The Typical American Diet

Today, the typical American diet consists primarily of feedlot beef, poultry, pork, and starchy foods like refined potato and corn products, white grains (like flour and rice), cereals, and hundreds of different processed, refined foods. Feedlot dairy products and eggs are also consumed on a regular basis. Our intake of sugar, approximately 150 pounds per person a year, is higher than the comparable sugar intake anywhere else in the world! Fruits, vegetables, beans, lentils, and whole grains are consumed in moderation, at best. Fish and raw nuts are rarely eaten, except for peanut butter. Peanuts are not nuts and peanut butter is usually full of sugar! Our sources of fat are mostly derived from saturated animal fats (meat, dairy, and eggs) that have little or no omega-3 fats to contribute to the diet. Obviously, the American diet has many opportunities to improve. Fortunately, some progress has been made in recent years.

Progress

One clear example of progress is the food industry's voluntary removal of trans fats from foods, although some processed foods still contain them (check food labels for any hydrogenated oils). Some restaurants, especially fast food restaurants, continue to use trans fats, also. One of my personal favorites is that butter, if used in moderation, has made a comeback. I used to receive an evil look whenever I cooked or offered butter instead of margarine to my guests. I was not being a renegade on purpose, but I remembered that in 1978 my organic chemistry teacher taught me to use butter. He said that margarine was not natural—maybe even unhealthful—and I have never used it since that time. Organic butter is preferred because it comes from pasture-fed cows and is full of omega-3 fats. Also, these cows do not consume feed (mostly corn and soybeans) that is full of pesticides, which is important because butter concentrates pesticides, and organic butter contains no growth hormones or antibiotics.

Another important improvement has been the addition of other oils available on the market, such as canola, extra virgin olive oil, and flaxseed oil, along with more exotic oils like walnut, almond, sesame seed, coconut, and macadamia nut. A quick note: don't fall for the new margarines that declare that they are "excellent sources of omega-3 fats." Read their nutritional facts label and you will find that they are also full of trans fats, outweighing any benefit derived from the omega-3 fats.

One more example of the improving American diet that makes my mother shake her head in disbelief is the popularity of vegetarian diets. More and more people are becoming vegetarians every day without withering away! Nutritional research has shown that vegetarian diets are healthier than the meat-and-potato diet for a variety of health issues such as heart disease and type 2 diabetes—those pesky risk factors for AD. Considering the amount of overweight and obese people in the United States, it is clear that most of us need to change our dietary choices. It is vital for us to include more omega-3 fats, fruits, and vegetables in our diets. We need to consume fewer saturated animal fats, dairy products, white grains, and less sugar. It will be helpful to avoid eating food from fast-food restaurants or limit visits as much as possible. And for all those cooks out there: potatoes, carrots, and any other belowground vegetables are very good for you if they are cleaned but not peeled or deep-fried!

The All-Important Ratio

Another extremely important point about the Mediterranean diet that is not apparent is the omega-6/omega-3 fat-balance ratio, which is in the healthy range of 1:1 to 4:1. This 4:1 ratio means that for every four grams of omega-6 fat consumed, one gram of omega-3 fat needs to be consumed. Unfortunately, the American diet is typically in the range of 10:1 to 20:1. What are omega-6 fats and why is this ratio so important?

Omega-6 and Omega-3 Fats

Omega-6 is another essential polyunsaturated fatty acid that the body cannot make itself. This fat also makes biologically active compounds that regulate the blood and immune systems, but it has the opposite effect from that of the omega-3 fats, and for beneficial reasons. In general, the role of omega-6 fat derivatives in the immune system is to start the immune reaction when a problem is detected by promoting the inflammatory response. Omega-3 fat derivatives exhibit a counter reaction in that they slow down the inflammatory response so that the cells and tissues can repair and heal themselves. Further important examples of their opposing reactions is that omega-6 fats cause blood vessels to contract and omega-3 fats relax them; omega-6s cause the blood to clot and omega-3s thin the blood. These complicated sets of opposing biochemical actions are necessary for maintaining your health. To keep your body in top shape, you need to consume both types of these essential fatty acids in a well-balanced ratio. For optimum health, this ratio should be between 1:1 and 4:1 of omega-6 to omega-3 fats but not the 10:1 to 20:1 ratio that the typical American diet represents!

There are two major problems with this high omega-6 to omega-3 ratio in our nutrition. Carbohydrates and proteins are broken down during digestion into smaller parts, but fatty acids stay relatively intact. If you consume many more omega-6 fats than omega-3 fats, your body will have mainly omega-6s to work with. Why? Here is the first major problem with a 20:1 ratio: both omega-6 and omega-3 fats share the same enzymatic pathway to make their important biochemically active derivatives. The essential fatty acid that wins the pathway is the one present in the highest amount. In the case of excess omega-6 fats, your body is constantly stimulating your blood to clot, raising your blood pressure, and over-activating the pro-inflammatory part of your immune system, to name just a few of many activities.

To understand the next major problem, just imagine what is happening in your body when twenty of the omega-6 fats trigger inflammation (when trouble such as a foreign invader or a wound is perceived), while only one omega-3 fat is triggered to stop the inflammation and allow your body to heal. The inflammatory response literally builds on itself, unable to stop because there are not enough omega-3 fats to extinguish the reaction. This condition is termed "chronic inflammation." In trying to help the problem, the immune system perpetuates the pro-inflammatory response and keeps the body in a constant systemic inflammatory state. This excessive amount of omega-6 fat is considered to be at the root of many diseases, including some cancers, type 2 diabetes, heart disease, and some dementias like Alzheimer's disease.

One Big Fat Mess

How did the American diet get into this mess? Again, it goes back to the 1950s when farm animals were taken out of the pastures where they ate a natural diet of mostly grasses, which are high in omega-3 fats. The animals were placed in feedlots where the core diet consists of corn and soybean products, which are practically devoid of omega-3 fats. The feedlot issue is what started the organic pasture-fed meat and free-range poultry movement. There has been an increasing demand for farm animals to be fed natural diets that provide their natural fat ratios.

Another factor previously mentioned was the use of inexpensive vegetable oils such as corn oil and cottonseed oil. Those oils are full of omega-6 fats and devoid of omega-3 fats. Even soybean oil, which is considered healthful and is therefore used in many convenience foods, is excessively high in omega-6 fats without enough omega-3 fats to provide any health benefits. High amounts of omega-6 fats are insidiously used in our food nowadays, especially for the purpose of replacing the trans fats. Almost all processed snack foods contain either soybean oil, corn oil, or both. Even a simple can of cream of mushroom soup is comprised of corn, cottonseed, and/or soybean oils.

More Bad Fats

The fact that omega-6 fats interfere with omega-3 fat metabolism is not the only problem. Animal meat contains various types of saturated fats. Animals are full of another non-essential fatty acid called arachidonic acid (AA), which is part of the omega-6 family. Arachidonic acid also competes with the fat-sharing enzymes, with omega-3s losing out again. To add to our health demise, trans fats also interfere with omega-3 uptake since they behave just like saturated fats! To top it all off, both saturated animal fats and trans fats raise detrimental blood cholesterol levels in the low density lipoproteins (LDL) and lower the beneficial cholesterol in high density lipoproteins (HDL). It bears repeating that it is not the cholesterol in food that raises your cholesterol levels, but it is the amount of saturated animal fats, trans fats, and refined carbohydrates one consumes that raise your LDL cholesterol levels and lower your HDL cholesterol levels!

Maintain a Proper Ratio

Ultimately, achieving the amazing health benefits from omega-3 fats depends on maintaining a ratio of no higher than 4:1 of omega-6/omega-3 fats, lowering your saturated animal fat levels, and eliminating trans fats from your diet. This balance keeps your blood pressure normal, your heartbeat regular, your blood vessels elastic, your immune system functioning at its best, and your complex brain operating smoothly. Once you are committed to maintaining the correct omega fats ratio, it will take anywhere from six months to a year for your body to reflect your improved dietary intake and to gain the heart and brain protection provided by this ratio.

More Good Fats

Olive oil is another important feature in the Mediterranean diet. It is not the key protective factor it was once thought to be, however, because it contains almost no omega-3 fats. Olive oil is primarily a monounsaturated fatty acid called omega-9, which has other important benefits that differ from omega-3 fats. One benefit is that olive oil has almost no omega-6 fats. It is a good alternative to the other vegetable oils, as it lowers the body's omega-6 fat load. Purchase only "extra virgin olive oil," which means that the olives have been cold-pressed and are unrefined. If the bottle says merely "olive oil," it has been refined. Edgar Cayce's readings regularly suggested using pure olive oil in massages and for a variety of health concerns. He also recommended that consuming a small amount of olive oil daily would be beneficial. Science has now caught up with Cayce's ideas on many issues, the benefits of olive oil being among them. New research has shown that extra virgin olive oil contains an enzyme that has anti-inflammatory properties. The properties act much like nonsteroidal anti-inflammatory drugs (NSAIDs), such as aspirin and ibuprofen, by blocking the activity of COX-1 and COX-2 (Beauchamp, G.K., 2005). This anti-inflammatory enzyme has been named oleocanthal and may be responsible for some of the health benefits associated with the Mediterranean diet. Although it would take a great deal of olive oil to relieve a headache, a daily dose of approximately two ounces, taken consistently over time like a low dose of aspirin, might provide substantial health benefits linked to chronic inflammation.

Nuts

Macadamia nuts, cashews, and hazelnuts are predominantly comprised of monounsaturated fats. Therefore, they are not significant sources of omega-6 fats. The almond was a nut mentioned regularly by Edgar Cayce: " . . . the readings recommend 'three almonds a day' as a guard against cancer." (3515-1, Report #1) There is now evidence that it was the bitter almond that Cayce was suggesting, not the sweet almond that is consumed today. Nevertheless, these sweet almonds are very nutritious and digest the most easily of all nuts. Almonds and most other nuts are full of calcium, magnesium, and folate, which are all extremely beneficial nutrients for the body.

Oils from the Tropics

Another interesting family of oils that was shunned in the 1950s is that of tropical oils—palm and coconut oil—because they contain saturated fats. It is now recognized that saturated fats behave differently depending on the size of their carbon chains. Tropical oils contain mostly saturated fats, which are medium-chained saturated fats (6–10 carbons), compared to most of the saturated animal fats, which are long chains (12-24 carbons). Their composition matters because these medium chains are not converted to cholesterol or placed into fat storage; instead, they are always used directly for energy. Palm oil is also a good source of vitamin E. Coconut oil, with the highest amount of medium-chained fatty acids, is especially beneficial for athletes and growing children. Most importantly, both do not contribute to heart disease because of their medium-chained fatty acid content, and they do not contain cholesterol. Since coconut oil contains 92 percent saturated fat, it can be stored for a long time at room temperature (and even longer in the refrigerator). It may be used for baking or stir-frying because it can take high heat without oxidizing. Health food markets sell it unrefined and with or without the coconut scent.

Another reason to consider using butter is that it also contains a significant amount of the medium-chained saturated fatty acids. If it is organic from pasture-fed cows, then it is truly healthful. Organic butter will contain more omega-3 fats along with no pesticides, growth hormones, or antibiotics, unlike regular butter.

Replace the Bad with the Good

Fish, nuts, and seeds—all high in omega-3 fats—as well as olive oil and all the other healthful oils mentioned, should *replace* other "bad' fats in the diet to achieve optimal health benefits. The goal is to decrease saturated animal fats, eliminate trans fats, and increase the omega-3 fats in our diets. Eating a handful of walnuts or flaxseeds while continuing to consume a diet high in saturated animal fats does not remove the health risk. If your total caloric intake of fat is in the healthy range, your diet may remain the same. It is the type of fat that must be changed in many diets. Consuming fish once a week or a vegetarian meal two to three times a week will displace meals that might be high in saturated animal fats. Eating this way is also one secret to weight loss because only saturated animal fats and trans fats (as well as an excess of glucose) go into those fat storage adipose cells!

Researchers have studied the relationship between eating fish and the resulting mental performance in a large group of middle-aged men and woman. Those who consumed a high percentage of their fat from fish had a low risk of mental decline, and those whose overall fat intake was high had a higher risk of mental decline. When these researchers looked at overall fat intake versus saturated animal fat intake, they found a *significant* relationship between a diet high in saturated animal fat and mental decline (Kalmijn, S., et al., 2004). There are two important messages here. The first message is that a balanced, nutritious low-fat diet in which most of the fat calories are from omega-3 fats and in which saturated animal fats are limited protects and might actually help prevent many diseases of the brain, such as dementia. The second point is that a diet high in saturated animal fat consumed during middle age caused mild declines in mental performance in people long before the symptoms of AD occurred.

Another related report in the journal *Neurology*, published in March 2008, looked at health exams done from 1964 to 1973 on 6,583 people who were forty to forty-five years old at the time of the exam and the subsequent incidence of AD in those people approximately thirty-six years later (Whitmer, R., et al., 2008). The risk of dementia for overweight and obese people was greatly increased because their risk of developing type 2 diabetes, heart disease, and stroke—all precursors of AD—was already high. Additionally, what this work showed was a new and separate risk factor, high belly fat! As part of the exam performed when they were in their early forties, their bellies were measured from the back to the upper abdomen. Above ten inches was considered high. Doctors now measure your waist circumference to determine high belly fat. The measurement is taken at the level of the belly button. For a man, a waist measurement greater than forty inches and for a woman, greater than thirty-five inches is considered high. It turned out that the larger the belly in midlife, the more likely the person was to develop dementia and AD later in life.

Even people possessing a normal body weight but a high belly measurement had a significantly increased risk for dementia. Researchers have learned that belly fat gives off a hormone called leptin that travels to the brain and regulates not only hunger and weight but also brain development and memory. Leptin is a neuroprotector, among other functions. As with insulin, the problem is that the receptors in the brain for leptin may become leptin-resistant in people with high belly fat. Even though having high belly fat does not cause AD, it does indicate that a person's health in early middle age might affect the risk of developing dementia and AD later in life. This correlation highlights the importance of making healthful dietary choices, starting NOW!

Simple Ideas to Improve Your Diet

Another example of the urgency to consume a healthier diet by adding more "good fats" into the diet is a study that tested whether omega-3 supplements could help people that already had mild to moderate symptoms of Alzheimer's disease. Unfortunately, the study showed that the supplements had no effect *except* on those people in the study possessing the mildest mental decline at the beginning of the study. These people had a far lower rate of decline in mental function at the end of the study than similarly functioning people who took a placebo (Freund-Levi, Y., et al., 2006). The salient point worth repeating is to protect your brain, and start *now!* Keep in mind that you do not need a daily supply of omega-3 fats; just maintain a weekly intake of around six to eight grams once you have brought your omega-6 fats down to that ratio between 1:1 and 4:1 omega-6/omega-3.

Here are some simple ideas to increase the use of omega-3 fats. Use flaxseed oil with red wine vinegar or balsamic vinegar on salads. These vinegars are nutritious, but don't use white vinegar, which is better for housecleaning. Dip sourdough or whole-grain bread into a mixture of olive oil and flaxseed oil. Pesto may be made with walnuts, basil, and olive oil and used in a variety of ways (both walnuts and basil contain omega-3 fats). Eat a handful of walnuts for an easy snack and add wheat germ or freshly ground flaxseed to your morning cereal or oatmeal. When baking homemade cookies and breads, substitute one-fourth of a cup of freshly ground flaxseed for one-fourth of a cup of flour. A quick note about the use of oils: never use flaxseed oil or extra virgin olive oil in sautéing or stir-frying, as they do not tolerate high heat. Instead, use butter or a mixture of butter and canola oil. If you are feeling adventurous, try using coconut oil or macadamia nut oil. Coconut oil is useful for cooking because of its high, medium-chained saturated fat content, as previously discussed. Macadamia nut oil is also effective for cooking because it can tolerate high heat (380°F) without breaking down or oxidizing, it has a long shelf life, and it is 80 percent monounsaturated fat. That is better than olive oil, and macadamia nut oil has almost no omega-6 fats, as a bonus!

Eat Nuts

Another interesting study in support of the Mediterranean diet revealed that consuming a diet high in nuts—especially walnuts—and fiber may lower your cholesterol even more efficiently than following a low-fat diet, which is the approach suggested in place of taking statin medication. The people who had the high nut and fiber diet reduced their LDL cholesterol levels by 13 percent, while the people on the low-fat diet only reduced their LDL cholesterol levels by 3 percent (Weingartner, Bohm, and Laufs, 2011). So, enjoy a handful of nuts and don't worry about the fat content. They are a source of good fats and nutrients.

Eat Fish and Vegetables

As the Mediterranean diet suggests, fish is now considered brain food. Studies have shown that people who ate fish as little as once a week exhibited a much lower rate of AD than those who rarely ate fish (Barberger-Gateau, P., et al., 2002). Interestingly, this same study also indicated a trend towards a delay of the onset of dementia in vegetarians. Consuming more vegetarian meals is a good dietary choice because if everyone started eating fish more than once a week, it might deplete our already-low supply of world fish. Try to consume sustainable fish in order to keep our oceans balanced and full of fish. The Monterey Bay Aquarium has a Web site that guides you to the best choices, and it is montereybayaquarium.org/seafoodwatch. If you have decided to adopt a vegetarian diet, cannot consume fatty types of fish on a regular basis, or just do not like the taste of fish, take a high-quality fish oil supplement and/or a flaxseed oil supplement three days a week, or more. Algae oil is an alternative to fish oil because algae are what give fish their omega-3 fats. Check with your doctor first before taking these supplements, especially if you are taking a blood-thinning medication. If you are worried about the toxins in fish oil, www.comsumerlab.com reported in 2004 that high-quality fish oil capsules did not contain mercury or other toxins. Nevertheless, it is always a good idea to check for a label that states that its fish oil is of the highest purity. My favorite way to increase my omega-3 fat consumption is to enjoy sushi or sashimi (raw fish with or without rice) at least once or twice a month. Not only is raw fish full of omega-3 fats, but the roe (fish eggs) and the seaweed wraps are, too. I would highly recommend the sea eel (not fresh water eel, for they are endangered), which has one of the highest contents of omega-3 fats, pound for pound, than any other food!

The important points in this chapter are:

1. Consume less meat and limit the consumption of processed meats.
2. Consume more vegetarian meals; strive for twice or three times a week or more.
3. Consume more fresh nuts, seeds, and ground flaxseed meal.
4. Have a meal of sustainable fish once a week, eat sushi or sashimi once a month, and/or take fish oil and flaxseed capsules three times or more a week.
5. Consume more fruits, vegetables, and whole grains, and eliminate the white grains.
6. Strive for an omega-6/omega-3 ratio between 1:1 and 4:1.
7. Consume organic, free-range meat, poultry, dairy products, and eggs, all of which preserve their natural, healthy fat ratio.
8. Consume only healthful oils like canola, flaxseed, olive, macadamia nut, walnut, and organic butter.
9. Stop eating foods from fast-food restaurants or limit those meals to once every two weeks.

4
~

Flaxseeds

Is the current publicity about flaxseeds warranted? What are the nutritional differences between flaxseeds and fish? The first difference is that flaxseed contains a plant-based omega-3 fat with no cholesterol, and fish contains an animal-based omega-3 fat with cholesterol. Flaxseeds have a total fat content of 41 percent, and this total can be broken down to approximately 19 percent omega-3, 10 percent mono-unsaturated, 8 percent omega-6, and 4 percent saturated fatty acids. The seeds consist of approximately 20 percent protein and have a total of 28 percent fiber, with 18 percent of that being insoluble and 10 percent being soluble fiber. We will find out why the fiber content is important later.

Fish

Fish does not contain any fiber but is a great protein source—salmon contains approximately 27 percent protein. Let's look at the makeup of a different popular fatty fish, the halibut. For a four-ounce serving of baked halibut fillet, the protein content is around 26 percent, and the total fat is approximately 3 percent. Of that 3 percent total fat, 1.4 percent is polyunsaturated, 0.9 percent is monounsaturated, and 0.7 percent is saturated. The fillet will have about forty-six milligrams of cholesterol.

Fish Versus Flaxseeds

Why was polyunsaturated fat used in the fish example while omega-3 and omega-6 fats were used in the flaxseed example? Polyunsaturated is a broad term that includes a variety of fatty acids that have more than one double bond in their chemical structure, which accommodates their various important functions. Omega-3 and omega-6 fats are technically known as polyunsaturated fatty acids. They are deemed "essential fatty acids" because our body requires them but cannot produce them from other fatty acids. In the case of the halibut, the 1.4 percent polyunsaturated fatty acid can be further broken down into 1 percent omega-3 and 0.4 percent omega-6. Salmon has about 4 percent polyunsaturated fatty acids, which can be broken down to 3.5 percent omega-3 and 0.5 percent omega-6.

Omega-3 and Omega-6 Families

To explain the other differences between flaxseed and fish, a larger view of these two essential fatty acids is necessary. Omega-3 and omega-6 are terms that refer to the occurrence of the first double bond of the fatty acid and actually include a number of polyunsaturated fatty acids in their respective families; highlighted next are the important ones.

Omega-6 was the first family to be identified, and its primary member is known as linoleic acid (LA). By adding double bonds, LA is then converted to gamma-linolenic acid (GLA) and then into arachidonic acid (AA). The next step in this conversion is where aspirin and other NSAIDs block the pathway, AA to cyclooxygenase-2 (COX-2). Here is the omega-6 family pathway, simplified:

$$LA \rightarrow GLA \rightarrow AA \rightarrow COX\text{-}2$$

In the omega-3 family, alpha-linolenic acid (ALA) is the primary member. ALA can be converted through a series of steps to eicosapentaenoic acid (EPA) and then to docosahexaenoic acid (DHA). Here is the omega-3 family pathway simplified:

$$ALA \rightarrow EPA \rightarrow DHA$$

None of these polyunsaturated fats is an end product, and the body uses all fats in a variety of ways. GLA, AA, and EPA fats have other pathways that generate end products, which, as a whole, are called eicosanoids. Eicosanoids are hormone-like molecules that are responsible for an enormous variety of different functions in your body. Some examples would be the ones previously discussed including the immune response, inflammation or anti-inflammation, and blood vessel constriction or relaxation. Depending on the pathway that generated them, these molecules are classified as prostaglandins, thromboxanes, or leukotrienes, and literally hundreds of these molecules have been identified by scientists to date.

Back to Flaxseed and Fish

Now back to flaxseed and fish. Flaxseed's total fat content is 41 percent, and of this total, 19 percent is the omega-3 fat ALA and 8 percent is the omega-6 fat LA. Flaxseeds and all plants have ALA omega-3 fats, which will be only partially converted to EPA and then to DHA. Of the 19 percent ALA in flaxseeds, approximately 2 percent is converted to EPA and only 0.5 percent to DHA. Fish contain EPA and DHA omega-3 fats, which are the most important fatty acids for the brain. Another reason to avoid a high omega-6 fat diet is that it can reduce the plant conversion of ALA to EPA and DHA by 40 percent because of the enzyme-sharing predicament mentioned previously.

Also needed for an optimum conversion of the omega-3 family is a diet containing plenty of vitamins B_6 and B_{12}. Folate, another B vitamin, increases the brain's concentration of EPA and DHA (Das, U., 2008). Fatty fish has a very different omega-3 composition. Salmon, with its total fat content of 11 percent, is broken down to 0.5 percent omega-6, 0.01 percent ALA, 0.5 percent EPA, and 3 percent DHA. As described earlier, EPA is important because it generates eicosanoids, which have effects throughout the body and are important for the structure and function of all the body's cell membranes. DHA is also found in the cell membranes throughout our bodies, but its highest concentration is in our brain and eyes. The brain requires a high amount of DHA in its membranes to perform the rapid firing of chemicals across the synapses of the neurons to communicate and carry out the brain's amazing array of functions. The retinas of our eyes also have a high demand for DHA to maintain good health.

Fish or Flaxseeds?

Why not simply eat fish instead of flaxseeds? Both are recommended as part of a nutritious diet because of several different issues. To receive the health benefits of omega-3 fats from fish, two meals a week consisting of a fatty fish are necessary, but that does not include shrimp, crab, lobster, red snapper, orange roughy, tilapia, or any farm-raised fish. There are two problems with these meals. First is the risk of heavy metal contamination, which is toxic to the entire body and compounds the effects of Alzheimer's disease on the brain. The second problem is that it would be environmentally foolish to recommend that everyone increase fish consumption to those levels, considering that worldwide fish stocks are already rapidly diminishing. Flaxseeds provide an excellent alternative. They are very nutritional and easy to grow, requiring hardly any water. For those very reasons, people have been consuming flaxseeds for centuries. To your daily diet, simply add two tablespoons of ground flaxseed meal, or one teaspoon of flaxseed oil, to receive the health benefits of omega-3 fats. Along with daily flaxseed consumption, go ahead and enjoy eating fish once a week to twice a month.

Other Good Sources of Omega-3 Fats

Include regularly in your diet the new high-DHA omega-3 egg, as this kind of egg contains as much EPA and DHA fat as three ounces of salmon. Dine on free-range, pasture-fed beef, lamb, and poultry, which are higher in omega-3 fats and contain fewer omega-6 fats than feed-lot animals. Keep in mind that the dairy products from pasture-fed cows (and goats) are higher in omega-3 fats, too! Additional sources of omega-3 fats are pumpkin seeds, wheat germ, and walnuts. There are other good sources not widely known because they are not considered to be high-fat foods, and the little fat they do contain is high in omega-3s. These include broccoli, cantaloupe, cauliflower, chard, Chinese cabbage, grape leaves, kale, kidney beans, parsley, spinach, and wheatgrass.

Changing the Ratio

An extremely important factor in optimizing the assimilation of omega-3 fats into the body is the necessary *elimination* of the high amounts of omega-6 fats that most of us consume today (Erasmus, U., 1993). It will take diligence and a great deal of food label reading until we have learned what products are acceptable, depending on our own specific diets. Eliminating as much as possible of omega-6 fats from all diets should be the first priority! This elimination can be accomplished by avoiding margarine, shortening, and any oils that are refined and not sold in dark or opaque bottles. Avoid any products that contain corn oil, cottonseed oil, or soybean oil. Additionally, avoid other refined oils in products such as mayonnaise, salad dressings, soups, and many other processed foods, especially snack foods. Avoid all commercial (feedlot) meats, dairy products, and eggs, as well as all processed meats and sausages. Limit the pasture-fed meat, organic dairy products, and the new omega-3 eggs for the first three to six months of your new diet in order to lower your omega-6 intake. After that time, enjoy those foods a few times a week, or in the case of organic butter, in moderation.

Give Your New Diet Three Weeks

The most exciting part of making this vital change is that it will only take about three weeks for your body to significantly increase the concentration of omega-3 fats in its tissues and for omega-6 fat concentrations to decrease. Depending on the size of your body, it should take approximately six to eight months to have omega-3 fats completely infused into your body's cells in order to receive the protective health benefits. After this time period, a diet comprised of a 4:1

ratio of omega–6 to omega–3 fats may be observed. If it appears difficult to calculate how much of one fat or another you need to achieve
this ratio, simply consume a natural, wholesome diet. This ratio is how
people used to eat before the industrial age. At that time, all farm
animals were pasture–fed and free–range, whole grains and cold-
pressed oils were the norm, processed, refined foods were nonexistent
(except for by the very wealthy), and most people had a garden for
growing fresh vegetables and fruit. The 4:1 ratio has been proven to be
beneficial by many cultures throughout time. It maintains a healthful
balance, and life is all about balance. In fact, the most important thing
you can do for your overall health is to keep yourself balanced spiri-
tually, mentally, and physically. One of Edgar Cayce's most enduring
quotes from the readings is " . . . for the spirit is life; the mind is the
builder; the physical is the result . . . "! (349-4)

The Importance of Fiber

Flaxseeds are important for another reason—fiber! With our increasingly busy lives, refined and packaged foods have made cooking and
eating easier but at a sacrifice to our health. Most of these items have
been stripped of their fiber. As a consequence, the typical American
consumes only from ten to twenty grams of fiber per day when the
optimal fiber amount is thirty to forty grams! Everyone needs to consume more fiber to achieve the perfect balance of assimilation and
elimination. Balancing food assimilation and elimination is a concept
that the Cayce readings regarded as the key to perfect health. What
occurs inside every cell in our body depends on what nutrients the
cell receives and how efficient it is at eliminating its waste products.

Soluble and Insoluble Fiber

There are two types of fiber that have important functions in our
bodies—soluble and insoluble fiber. Soluble fiber dissolves in fluids to
form a gel, thus helping to soften stools and assist in their elimination.
Insoluble fiber is insoluble in fluids, but it soaks up fluids like a sponge,
also. With this swelling action, it acts as a bulking agent, accelerating
the time fecal waste transits the lower bowels. Assimilation of nutri-

ents is increased with a fiber-rich meal because the food is processed more slowly through the upper digestive tract as the fiber is broken down, but not digested, so that the nutrients are slowly released. Flaxseeds have both soluble and insoluble fiber at a rate of 2.5 grams of total fiber per tablespoon.

Lignans

Flaxseeds have another fiber trick up their sleeves—lignans. Of all foods, flaxseeds have the highest amount of lignans, and they are also one of the only foods to contain a significant amount. Berries such as strawberries and blackberries also contain lignans, as do nuts, beans, and whole grains, but flaxseeds possess much higher levels.

Lignans are phytochemicals that have many biological activities in the body. Lignans from flaxseeds demonstrate strong anti-inflammatory actions by helping to block the pro-inflammatory actions so that cellular repair can begin. They also have strong antioxidant properties. In addition to containing vitamins C and E, one important property of lignans is protecting the LDL's cholesterol from being oxidized by free radicals as it travels through the bloodstream. LDL makes cholesterol available to the cells of all the body's tissues and organs, including the brain. One study even links oxidized cholesterol, not un-oxidized or healthful cholesterol, with increased neuronal damage as seen in AD (Gamba, P., et al., 2011). Lignans and other phytochemicals, along with other antioxidants, are the body's main damage control team. Holding oxidant damage to a minimum protects your whole body, especially your arteries, heart, and brain, by lowering systemic inflammation and keeping your body in optimum condition.

Add Fiber

How does fiber relate to Alzheimer's disease? Fiber lowers blood cholesterol, which reduces the risk of heart disease and helps normalize blood glucose and insulin levels. This normalization in turn reduces the risk of type 2 diabetes. Both heart disease and diabetes are known risk factors for AD. Another product that might help with these two conditions was recommended by the Cayce readings—steel cut oats for breakfast. Steel cut oats are healthier than regular oatmeal because of how they are processed. If you already have type 2 diabetes, a high–fiber diet reduces your body's insulin demand because of the gradual release of glucose from the fiber into the blood stream. This diet not only includes the obvious whole grain foods like oats, brown rice, barley, wheat, and flaxseed, but also contains fruits and vegetables. Most fruits and vegetables contain a balance of soluble and insoluble fiber, and especially high in fiber are apples, beans, and peas.

How to Include Flaxseeds in Your Diet

There are plenty of ways to include flaxseeds in your diet. Use a mixture of flaxseed oil and extra virgin olive oil in salad dressings; mix a tablespoon of ground flaxseed with honey and spread it on toast; sprinkle ground flaxseed on cereal, yogurt, salads, or soups; and mix ground flaxseed into meatloaf, meatballs, or hamburgers (using pasture–fed meat, of course). It is also easy to add ground flaxseed to the batter of pancakes, muffins, cookies, or other baked goods (another hint is to use one-fourth less sugar in these recipes). Why use only ground flaxseed? Because whole flaxseeds will pass directly through your digestive tract undigested. Purchase whole flaxseeds and grind them yourself in a coffee grinder or buy ground flaxseed meal in vacuum–packed bags. Store both of them in the refrigerator to prevent their oils from oxidizing. Whole flaxseeds will last a year, while ground flaxseed will last about four months. You will notice in a grocery or health food store that there are two types of flaxseeds—a reddish brown type and a golden brown type. Their taste is a little different, but nutritionally they are the same. If you buy flaxseed oil, make sure it is from the refrigerated section of the store and that it has the lignans added back into it. Store this oil in the refrigerator, also, or in your freezer for longer storage.

Points to remember from this chapter:
1. Add more ground flaxseed meal and flaxseed oil to your diet.
2. Start on a program to eliminate omega–6 fats from your diet for six to eight months.

3. Consume more omega-3 fats to achieve a balance ratio of 4:1 omega-6 to omega-3 fats.

4. Add more fiber into your diet for better assimilation and elimination, which are the keys to health.

5
~

Real Fruits and
Vegetables Do Matter

There are various theories about the pathology of Alzheimer's disease (AD), and recent evidence supports the hypothesis that oxidative stress caused by inflammation occurs early in the progression of the disease. All the large molecules in the brain—lipids, proteins, nucleic acids (DNA and RNA)—and even sugars are affected by oxidation, leading to neuronal damage. Oxidation occurs significantly before the senile plaques and neurofibrillary tangles develop, which are the hallmarks of the disease. Some researchers have taken this hypothesis a step further, suggesting that the purpose of the initial development of the β-amyloid protein and the phosphorylated tau is to combat oxidative damage and keep the neurons healthy (Moreira, P., et al., 2008). However, as oxidative stress accelerates, the antioxidant activity of each agent may be overwhelmed. Then, as the neurons are damaged beyond repair, the β-amyloid protein aggregate becomes the plaques and tau hyperphosphorylates. This action causes the tangles, which may result in more oxidation, thus leading to dementia and AD (Castellani, R., et al., 2008).

Whole Foods

How can we manage oxidation so that the damage does not occur in the first place, and how can we reverse any damage that has already occurred? A healthful diet can decrease inflammation. A decrease in inflammation keeps oxidative stress under control and allows the body to heal. The ability to reduce oxidative stress demonstrates that what you currently consume in your diet appears to be one thing you *can* do to lower your risk for AD and enjoy your life in great health and in full control (Bonda, D., et al., 2010).

Maintaining the health of your brain is as simple as adding whole foods and emphasizing antioxidants in your diet. The term "whole foods" simply means that the food is still whole, as Mother Nature produced it. Apples are an example of a whole food, but once they are processed into apple juice, applesauce, dried apples, or any other re-fined apple product, they are no longer a whole food. Fresh apple juice or any other apple products are not necessarily bad for you; they just do not have the apple's entire set of nutrients since many are lost during processing. The term "whole foods" does not imply the con-sumption of only raw foods; instead, it represents the opposite of pro-cessed and refined foods. Lightly cooked vegetables, baked or mashed potatoes with their skins intact, cooked beans, and steel–cut oatmeal, to give a few examples, are still considered whole foods. Grains like brown rice, barley, quinoa, oats, wheat, and rye are still whole when they are milled in their entirety, which removes only the husk and leaves the original kernel intact. Refining grains to make products like white flour and white rice involves stripping away the bran and the germ of the kernel where most of their nutrients reside. Also, beware of products that claim to be made of wheat flour, which is actually white flour with a little bit of bran mixed in. To qualify as a whole food, the label must state that the product is made of whole grain wheat. Nuts and seeds still in their shells are also good choices. Quick-frozen fruits and vegetables are also acceptable. Free–range animals like chickens and turkeys, pasture–fed beef, pork, lamb, and wild-caught fish are considered to be whole foods because *they* consume the diet that Mother Nature originally provided for them.

Phytochemicals

When we consume whole foods, we receive dozens of vitamins and minerals and hundreds of other nutrients. In the case of plants, we also consume thousands of non-nutrient compounds that all work together in relatively unknown ways to influence our bodies. These multiple interactions are unknown because scientists can only study one compound at a time in the laboratory. Scientists isolate a single compound to see how it reacts within a given set of rules that are already known. This process is *not* how our bodies and the foods we consume go about their activities! The interactions of nutrients and non-nutrient compounds work synergistically in our bodies, which is constantly changing and adapting to our environment.

Phytochemicals in Food

We are all familiar with vitamins and minerals, but what are these other nutrients and non-nutrients that are running around in our bodies? The "other nutrients" are proteins, fiber, carbohydrates, and fats. The "non-nutrients" are the phytochemicals mentioned earlier. They are considered non-nutrients because our bodies could function without them, but we are far better off with them when it comes to disease prevention. Importantly, phytochemicals are only found in plants. Berries have the most phytochemicals, with blueberry in the lead at over 15,000. Broccoli has as many as 10,000 different ones, the lowly pinto bean has almost 12,000, and a potato with its skin intact has almost 5,000!

Even coffee, with or without caffeine, is full of phytochemicals. A recent study showed that those who drank three to five cups of coffee per day in midlife were much less likely to develop dementia (Eskelinen, M., et al., 2009). Now, I understand why the Cayce readings regarded coffee as food, with the warning not to add milk or cream since this mixture does not digest very well. Nutritionists have learned that the milk and cream bind with some phytochemicals, and so they are not assimilated. Tea—especially green tea—dark chocolate, and red wine are also very healthful, possibly offering protection against AD as a consequence of their vast array of phytochemicals!

Plants Are Important

These amazing phytochemicals are found in every plant—including whole grains, legumes (beans and lentils), nuts, fruits, vegetables, and herbs. Each plant has its own phytochemical makeup, providing specific tastes, aromas, colors, and other unique characteristics. Phytochemicals from plants play a multitude of different roles in our bodies. They function as antioxidants and as metal chelators, and many have disease-inhibiting abilities. Some even mimic certain hormones in our bodies. Only a fraction of the tens of thousands of compounds are known. The largest class is called flavonoids, with over 5,000 identified by researchers so far. The higher the intake of phytochemicals (and flavonoids in particular) that you consume, the less risk you have of developing dementia (Commenges, D., et al. 2000).

There are many other classes of phytochemicals that have been identified, such as carotenoids, capsaicins, polyphenols, and phytosterols, to name just a few. Five of the popularly known ones cited for health benefits in recent years are lycopene from tomatoes; lutein from leafy greens and fruits; resveratrol from grapes, berries, and peanuts; lignans from flaxseeds; and quercetin from apples, onions, and garlic. Even though many of these phytochemicals have been isolated and are now sold as supplements, the way that they interact with the other thousands of phytochemicals to bring about their health benefits is unknown. There might be risks in taking these isolated phytochemicals in high doses, and in some cases it may even be dangerous! For example, resveratrol in megadoses (more than 300 mgs) increases the risk for lymphoma in humans. Lymphoma is a cancer that originates in a type of white blood cell called a lymphocyte (Papp, K., 2007). One would be wiser to consume a wide variety of whole foods in generous quantities to gain all of the amazing benefits that these phytochemicals have to offer.

The Role of Antioxidants

Let's have an overview of antioxidants to understand why they are vital to our well-being. The principal role of antioxidants is to inactivate free radicals. Antioxidants donate an electron to the free radical, which inactivates or stops the radical from damaging the cells in your body. Free radical damage is thought to be a major cause of aging in general, and it plays a key role in dementia. These unstable and highly reactive free radicals are produced naturally in the body and also by external agents such as infections, cigarette smoke, drugs, herbicides, pesticides, pollutants, toxins, and radiation from the sun. Given that the brain *naturally* produces more free radicals than any other organ in your body (because of its high-energy needs) while producing the lowest amount of natural antioxidants, it is very important to consume plenty of antioxidants to reduce the damage. Even though antioxidants have a primary role to perform, they are a diverse group. Many antioxidants play different roles other than inactivating free radicals. This group includes some vitamins; most notable are vitamins C and E, some minerals such as selenium, and a multitude of phytochemicals.

The Wonders of Vitamin C

Vitamin C (ascorbic acid) is number one in this group for its various roles. First, vitamin C is one of the most important antioxidants in our line of defense against disease since it is water-soluble. It is therefore found in the intercellular (between the cell) and intracellular (inside the cell) fluids of the entire body. The new vitamin C supplement called Ester-C is both water- and fat-soluble. These attributes mean that the vitamin C can go into the cell's membrane to attack free radicals there, as well as in all of the cellular fluids. Ester-C also stays in the body four times longer than the water-soluble type of vitamin C because it is fat-soluble. Ester-C is a supplement that most doctors and nutritionists recommend since we cannot get it from foods. The brain's high-energy rate from our thinking and processing requires a large amount of oxygen, making vitamin C extremely important to its function.

These biological reactions involving oxygen naturally generate a multitude of free radicals called "reactive oxygen species" (ROS). The fact that the membranes of neurons are rich in polyunsaturated fatty acids that are highly vulnerable to ROS damage helps us to understand why the brain tries to keep high concentrations of vitamin C available to it, especially compared with the rest of the body. Vitamin C also works within all cells to protect their components from free radical oxidation. This work is especially true for proteins. Protein oxidation may cause the proteins to stick together and aggregate, rendering them nonfunctional, and this process may also contribute to aging. Remember the "advanced glycation end products" (AGEs)? These free radicals have been found in the brain lesion of AD patients (Sanchez-Moreno and Martin, 2006). AGEs occur when a protein is oxidized. When the blood glucose levels are high, the oxidized protein is cross-linked with a sugar. Vitamin C not only protects the proteins from being oxidized but also stops the AGEs in their tracks, helping to prevent a chain reaction. Vitamin C is a very important cofactor for several enzymatic reactions; in the brain this reaction involves the formation of neurotransmitters such as dopamine and norepinephrine. Vitamin C may also act as a scavenger by helping the brain dispose of heavy metals like lead, mercury, copper, and environmental toxins. The lack of vitamin C weakens arteries and other tissues because vitamin C is necessary to make collagen and elastin. Collagen and elastin preserve the strength of arteries and tissues and also protect the skin from wrinkles.

The Brain's Immune System

The brain's immune system must react swiftly to an invader like bacteria or a virus because the neurons are highly vulnerable to damage. Remember that the immune system's first line of defense to an invader is the phagocytes, those specialized cells that release a "respiratory burst" of reactive oxygen in the form of hydroxyl made from hydrogen peroxide. A high concentration of vitamin C is needed to quickly reduce, or give electrons to, the reactive oxygen released in the "respiratory burst." Otherwise, the extra oxygen that did not hit and kill the invader will damage the brain's neurons. Along the lines of offense are the brain's astrocytes. Like microglia, they are essential to the functioning of the brain's immune system because they clean up debris from metabolism and invaders. Astrocytes also provide the neurons with important nourishment to maintain proper function. Human astrocytes grown in a petri dish that were supplemented with vitamin C increased in concentration and had their many functions enhanced (Martin, Joseph, and Cuervo, 2002).

There have been several studies that have investigated the role of vitamin C relative to mental performance and found a positive association, with low levels of vitamin C correlating to low memory performance (Deschamps, V., et al., 2001). Another study reviewed patients with severe Alzheimer's disease, moderate AD, and no AD, as it measured their dietary intake and blood plasma levels of vitamin C. In patients with AD, blood plasma vitamin C levels decreased in proportion to the severity of mental decline, even though the intake of vitamin C for the entire group was similar. The researchers attributed this result to the brain's response related to combating oxidative stress in the patients with Alzheimer's disease (Riviere, S., et al., 1998). This study contributes even more evidence that an increased intake of fruits and vegetables, especially those with high concentrations of vitamin C, may reduce your risk of dementia and AD.

Vitamin E—The Defender

Vitamin E is a fat-soluble vitamin and is one of the body's main defenders against free radical damage to cell membranes and internal cell components. Vitamin E is found predominantly in nuts and seeds—especially almonds, hazelnuts (filberts), pine nuts, walnuts, and sunflower seeds. It is also in asparagus, avocados, barley, brown rice, oats, olives, spinach, wheat germ oil, and cold-pressed vegetable oils, especially palm oil. In their roles as antioxidants, vitamins E and C work in tandem to stop free radicals and especially to break destructive chain reactions that occur when free radicals become really radical. If there is a lack of antioxidants to stop these chain reactions, we have learned that oxidative stress can occur. Remember that oxidative stress means that the production of oxidants (free radicals) exceeds the body's ability to defend itself, causing cell and tissue damage over time. Vitamin E defends the body by donating an electron to a free radical and inactivating both of them. Then, vitamin C comes along and donates an electron to vitamin E, making it active again. During the rapid-fire formation of free radicals, which causes a chain reaction, vitamin C not only helps vitamin E but also donates electrons directly to the free radicals to stop the chain reaction as soon as possible.

Low concentration of vitamin E is frequently observed in patients with Alzheimer's disease, suggesting that supplementation in middle age might delay the development of dementia and AD. There is evidence that the use of vitamin E and C supplements in combination may significantly reduce the prevalence of Alzheimer's disease. One study showed the risk of developing AD decreased by 78 percent in the elderly population that took both supplements (Zandi, P., et al., 2004).

Most of us are familiar with only one kind of vitamin E, alpha-tocopherol, which is the main type used in supplements and in most scientific studies. In nature, there are eight different varieties of vitamin E—or isoforms—that have activity: four tocopherols (alpha, beta, gamma, and delta) and four tocotrienols (alpha, beta, gamma, and delta). All eight isoforms function effectively as antioxidants, yet they differ widely in their biological effects. A few examples are that both alpha- and gamma-tocopherols are found to reduce the LDL cholesterol and increase the HDL cholesterol: alpha-tocotrienol protects neurons against toxins, and gamma-tocotrienol is the most potent isoform for lowering total blood cholesterol levels. Current developments show that all four tocotrienols are powerful neuroprotectors and antioxidants, possessing anti-cancer and cholesterol-lowering properties (Sen, Khanna, and Roy, 2006).

The latest research investigated the association of all eight isoforms of vitamin E and the occurrence of AD. Scientists found that the neuroprotective effects were related to the combination of all eight different isoforms, and that these effects were associated with a reduced risk of Alzheimer's disease. Research also discovered that the only isolated form of vitamin E that was associated with a reduced risk of AD was beta-tocopherol. The protection offered by beta-tocopherol alone was not as significant as that given by the combination of all eight isoforms (Mangialasche, F., et al., 2010). Beta-tocopherol is found in most nuts and seeds, but hazelnuts (filberts) and sunflower seeds have the highest levels of any other foods. Unfortunately, it is almost impossible to get the amount of vitamin E that is needed for these healthful benefits in our diet, and so a supplement is recommended. Look for supplements that have mixed tocopherols (all four isoforms) in the range of 200 to 400 IUs. Supplements that include the four tocotrienols are harder to find, but with so much new research surfacing regarding their health benefits, they will soon be widely available. To include all eight members of the "family" and their phytochemicals, it would be wise to consume, along with the supplements, a variety of whole foods rich in vitamin E in order to receive the health advantages from this diverse group of vitamins.

Glutathione (GSH) — The Natural Antioxidant

The best antioxidant of all is glutathione (GSH), and our bodies make it naturally! Glutathione not only stops those damaging free radicals, but also removes all sorts of poisonous chemicals and toxins from our bodies before they can do any harm. GSH is a tripeptide (a peptide is a small protein) made from three amino acids, cysteine, glycine, and glutamic acid. The body also needs selenium to make GSH, which is one reason that selenium is considered an antioxidant. Selenium is found in seafood, meat, whole grains, Brazil nuts, and many vegetables. Sulfur is also needed to make GSH, but only vitamin B_1 (thiamine) and the amino acids cysteine and methionine contain sulfur. Eggs contain B_1 as well as both of these amino acids, which is another important reason to consume eggs on a regular basis. Other foods that contain sulfur are beans, Brussels sprouts, cabbage, garlic, kale, and onions.

Add More GSH

With our increasing twenty–first–century lifestyle demands, adding more of this little peptide GSH to our system will help us to remain healthy. GSH is found in almost every fruit and vegetable but is mostly destroyed by the cooking process. Try to eat many of these foods raw or just lightly cooked or steamed. Vegetables such as broccoli, cabbage, Brussels sprouts, cauliflower, kale, and parsley not only contain GSH, but they also have phytochemicals that naturally make our bodies produce more glutathione. Interestingly, fish oil also causes our body to produce more GSH, and vitamin C helps to boost GSH levels—demonstrating more examples of synergy.

Alpha Lipoic Acid

Another assistant is alpha lipoic acid, a powerful universal antioxidant in itself. Alpha lipoic acid helps to produce GSH and has the ability to recycle GSH along with vitamins C and E, making all of them more efficient at capturing free radicals. Alpha lipoic acid is considered universal because it is both water- and fat-soluble. This attribute means that, like Ester-C, it can fight free radicals from both outside and inside the cell as well as in between the membranes of every cell in our bodies. Alpha lipoic acid is a sulfur-containing fatty acid that is also essential for our mitochondria, which are the power plants in our cells. The body does make a small amount of alpha lipoic acid that is needed for the mitochondria to generate energy, but there is not much left over for producing GSH or for it to act as an antioxidant. We need more of this antioxidant as we age. Alpha lipoic acid has another unique property. It prevents glycation (when a protein cross-links with a sugar)–protecting all the proteins in our body. It also reverses glycation that has already occurred (Perricone, N., 2000). Taking this supplement is beneficial due to the extra free radical protection throughout the body. An amount between 100 and 200 milligrams is considered to be an ideal dose for maintaining good health (Pressman and Buff, 2007).

Our Mitochondria and Alzheimer's Disease: Acetyl-L-Carnitine

While we are on the subject, the mitochondria have also been implicated in the pathology of Alzheimer's disease, and one reason may be acetyl-L-carnitine. Acetyl-L-carnitine is a nutrient that is made in our bodies from the amino acids lysine and methionine, and vitamin C also aids in its production. Acetyl-L-carnitine's main role is to transport fat to the mitochondria to make energy. Low vitamin C levels lower acetyl-L-carnitine levels, making it harder for cells to convert fat into energy. Although the brain's main energy source is glucose, the rest of your body derives 40–45 percent of its energy from fat, which keeps you active and healthy. Acetyl-L-carnitine is an antioxidant, and it increases GSH, as well. Acetylcholine, the neurotransmitter that is essential to memory and is known to decline as the severity of AD increases, needs acetyl–L–carnitine to be produced. In double–blind controlled studies, this nutrient was reported to have beneficial effects on depression and AD (Pettegrew and McClure, 2002). There is no need to supplement with acetyl–L–carnitine as long as your protein intake is adequate, but it is very important to consume numerous fruits and vegetables containing vitamin C to increase the efficiency of acetyl–L–carnitine. There are supplements available that contain both acetyl–L–carnitine and alpha lipoic acid. These supplements may help to keep your mitochondria in tiptop shape and to provide plenty of antioxidants to your brain.

Coenzyme Q10

The mitochondria also require a vitamin–like, fat–soluble substance called coenzyme Q10 or Co–Q10. It is also called ubiquinone (from the word ubiquitous), because it is found everywhere in our bodies. It is necessary for basic cellular functions as a coenzyme. A coenzyme is needed by the cell's enzymes to become active so that they can perform their numerous tasks. Co–Q10, which is also found in high amounts in the mitochondria, is essential for energy production. The coenzyme is in our cell membranes where it serves as an antioxidant and a recycler of vitamin E. As an antioxidant, Co–Q10 greatly reduces oxidative damage to tissues in general and inhibits the oxidation of the LDL cholesterol as it travels through the arteries on the way to the tissues and cells for use. Co–Q10 is biosynthesized in our bodies from the amino acid tyrosine in a seventeen–step pathway that requires all of the B vitamins as well as some trace minerals.

Similar to many other substances made in the body, levels of Co–Q10 decline with age. After midlife, this pathway is not as efficient as it was before the age of thirty, when the body's natural Co–Q10 levels were adequate for energy production. Statin drugs and other cholesterol–reducing drugs that block the cholesterol pathway also block the body from making Co–Q10 since they use parts of the same pathway for biosynthesis (Whitaker, J., 2002). Coenzyme Q10 is found in almonds, ocean salmon, sardines, spinach, and red meat (especially beef hearts). Since it is almost impossible to get enough from diet alone in our later years, it is recommended that everyone over forty years of age take thirty to fifty milligrams of Co–Q10 daily. Because it is a natural substance, there has not been a great deal of research performed on the relationship between Co–Q10 and AD. One study on mice demonstrated that Co–Q10 and vitamin E taken together—not separately—improved their cognitive abilities (McDonald, Sohal, and Forster, 2005). It seems reasonable that a deficiency in Co–Q10 would increase the risk for AD, since it is impossible for any system—especially the brain with its considerable energy production—to function efficiently with a shortage of fuel from the mitochondria.

The B Vitamins

If getting plenty of antioxidants is not reason enough to stock up on whole foods to prevent many diseases including Alzheimer's disease, then perhaps understanding the B vitamins will motivate you! As with the phytochemicals, every B vitamin is dependent on every other B vitamin. They work synergistically with all of the other nutrients and phytochemicals. The main role of the B vitamins is to serve as coenzymes that facilitate the work of every cell in our body. Vitamin B_6 (pyridoxine), for example, is involved with over one hundred reactions, many having to do with neurotransmitters. Low levels of vitamin B_3 (niacin), vitamin B_6, vitamin B_{12} (methylcobalamin), and folic acid (folate is the natural form found in food) have all been implicated in dementia and heart disease. Studies show that a large number of senior citizens have general vitamin B shortages, especially B_1 (thiamin, the one with sulfur), B_6, B_{12}, and folate (Whitney and Rolfes, 2002). Long–term, moderate nutrient deficiencies may cause seniors to become depressed and forgetful, causing them to eat less and producing even more memory problems and confusion. They might move to a nursing home and eat institutional foods that are predominantly refined and processed, containing very few nutrients. Subsequently, these individuals might decline further and even be diagnosed with dementia. Although eating a variety of whole foods is a much better way to acquire the nutritive benefits that B vitamins have to offer, if you are over sixty years old, it is recommended to take a vitamin B–complex supplement. Remember to discuss taking any supplements with your doctor.

Niacin — Vitamin B₃

Let's go over the B vitamins that have implications in dementia and Alzheimer's disease. A deficiency in B_3 (niacin) has long been known to cause depression and memory loss. The latest research has found that niacin in a form called niacinamide protects the neurons themselves by stabilizing the microtubules and increasing the clearance and decreased accumulation of the hyperphosphorylated tau (Green, K., et al., 2008).

Foods high in niacin include meats, poultry, fish, eggs, peanuts, mushrooms, spinach, and whole grains. Naturally occurring niacin is preferable because supplementing niacin in high doses (over 1000 mgs) produces many adverse side effects. Most notable is the "niacin flush," which may be painful and cause liver damage. According to the researchers, however, taking a multivitamin or B-complex vitamin that includes niacinamide is safe and has no side effects. Most likely, these vitamins have enough niacin to protect your neurons. Since the original research studied mice, a human trial to find the optimum dosage of niacinamide was initiated in the fall of 2008.

Pyridoxine — Vitamin B₆

Vitamin B_6, with its involvement in over one hundred chemical reactions, is so vital to your body that a deficiency involves a general failure for all of the body's systems. Although true deficiencies are rare, B_6 is readily destroyed in food production, such as refining, canning, and freezing. Storage in your freezer also destroys pyridoxine. If there is any B_6 left after the processing or storage of food, the rest is lost in the cooking process. Up to a third of all senior citizens have low levels of B_6 (Whitney and Rolfes, 2002). Without adequate amounts of B_6, the various syntheses of key neurotransmitters diminish. Symptoms may include depression, irritability, and confusion. Family members may conclude that these symptoms are demonstrating the onset of AD, when what the senior member may actually need is a diet consisting of unprocessed, whole foods! Excellent B_6 sources are chicken, pork, beef, fish, dairy products, and eggs. On the plant side, good sources are avocados, bananas, broccoli, carrots, potatoes, spinach, squash, tomatoes, and watermelons.

Methylcobalamin—Vitamin B$_{12}$—And Folic Acid

Vitamins B$_{12}$ (methylcobalamin) and folate (folate occurs naturally in food, and folic acid is the synthetic form of this water-soluble vitamin) depend on each other for activation for use by the body. When folate is digested in your stomach, a methyl group (CH$_3$) is added, and then the folate in the inactive form is delivered to all the cells in your body. To activate folate for cell use, vitamin B$_{12}$ removes the methyl group and thus becomes active itself. Once these B vitamins are activated, they are ready for the DNA synthesis that is required by both of them, providing many other important pathways. Excellent sources of folate are all of the legumes (beans and lentils), asparagus, avocados, broccoli, citrus, eggs, okra, tomatoes, spinach, and all of the leafy green vegetables. Most of these foods are also excellent sources of vitamin C. Vitamin C prevents folate from being broken down in the body too quickly, which is important because we only absorb about half the folate we take in from food and supplements.

The sources of vitamin B$_{12}$ are almost exclusively found in foods derived from animals (meat, poultry, shellfish, dairy, and eggs). All mushrooms contain a small amount of vitamin B$_{12}$ because they are fungi–which are neither animal nor plant–but not enough B$_{12}$ for adequate intake, excluding all other sources. Mushrooms also contain numerous phytochemicals–with many acting as antioxidants–and have even more than some vegetables! Therefore vegans who exclude all foods from animal sources should take a vitamin B$_{12}$ supplement, and everyone should enjoy a variety of mushrooms. Another concern with B$_{12}$ is that it is completely destroyed by microwave heating.

In the case of vitamin B$_{12}$, most seniors are known to be deficient because of malabsorption and should take a supplement. The most absorbable form is *methyl*cobalamin. A sublingual supplement, which is taken under the tongue, is most effective because it goes directly into the blood stream. Sublingual vitamin B$_{12}$ is readily absorbed into the cells, and taking it three times a week is usually sufficient. This methyl form is far more expensive and is generally not found in B-complex or multivitamin supplements. The kind of B$_{12}$ that is called *cyano*cobalamin is less expensive to produce but is more difficult for the body to absorb. Very little of it is actually absorbed by the cells so that it is still possible to be deficient in B_{12} when taking cyanocobalamin (Balch, P., 2006).

Antacids and Acids

B_{12} and folate also share another issue, and it concerns antacids. In one study, researchers found that people who took antacids for more than two years had a decline in cognitive performance. The decline ranged from mild to potentially severe dementia (Boustani, M., et al., 2007). Antacids interfere with the absorption of B_{12} and folate, because both vitamins need the stomach's digestive acids in order to release them from foods. Taking an antacid neutralizes these digestive acids, perhaps soothing your stomach but also leaving much of your food undigested. Especially undigested are proteins and many nutrients, including vitamins B_{12}, folate, vitamin D, and vitamin E. These nutrients will simply go down the drain.

The stomach's digestive acids are also the first line of defense against microbes found in foods because the acid kills most of them. This defense might seem trivial, but having dangerous microbes in your body may be life threatening. One example, *Clostridium difficile* or C-diff, is a bacterium that has already caused many deaths and is fast becoming a worldwide epidemic. It has become more prevalent with the overuse of antibiotics and antacids. Another concern is the link between dangerous microbes and atherosclerosis, another risk factor for AD. The hypothesis is that these invader microbes are attacked by the immune system with oxygen through the "respiration burst," which may also damage the arteries. Under normal circumstances, enough antioxidants would take care of the problem. With thousands of microbes constantly streaming into the blood, the damage develops out of control. Oxidative stress and inflammation take over and eventually clog the arteries. Calcium, which is important for strong bones and proper nerve function, is also affected by antacids because it also needs an acidic environment to be absorbed. In addition, as we grow older, our own digestive acids diminish, making our absorption of many nutrients less than optimal.

Heartburn and Indigestion

People over sixty years of age will often benefit by taking a good digestive aid that has enzymes like amylase, protease, lipase, and cellulase, as well as enzymes from papaya (papain) and pineapples (bromelain). Those enzymes support natural digestion and may eliminate heartburn so that an antacid may not be needed. Other advice for reducing heartburn is to try slippery elm lozenges, which may be found in health food stores. The slippery elm product coats the throat and stomach, contains antioxidants that help relieve inflammation in the intestine, and boosts mucus production to protect the stomach. The smoke from cigarettes weakens the valve or sphincter that connects the throat with the stomach, so do quit smoking. Don't consume huge, complicated meals; keep it simple so that your digestive system is able to work as efficiently as possible. Do not eat dinner or any snacks two to three hours before going to bed, as sleep slows digestion. Also, being overweight may worsen unwanted symptoms.

Another way to reduce heartburn is to eat slowly and chew your food well—Edgar Cayce recommended chewing every mouthful fourteen times (595-1). Chewing slowly increases the surface area of the food material, allowing the digestive enzymes to work more efficiently. Drink as little fluid as possible during meals; fluids dilute the digestive enzymes, making them less effective. Drink fluids, preferably plenty of water, between meals. Another tip from the Cayce readings recommends not eating while angry or upset (303-41). (Remember, the stress hormone cortisol shuts down the digestive system.) So, eat simply, do not gulp down your food, and take plenty of time to experience your meals in a relaxed atmosphere with a grateful attitude.

Toxic Homocysteine

Homocysteine has received considerable interest recently because high levels may be particularly toxic to both the heart and the brain. Vitamins B_6, B_{12}, and folate are especially important B vitamins that participate in the recycling, or if necessary the breakdown, of homocysteine. These three vitamins work together to keep this key biochemical pathway running smoothly. When one of these B vitamins is low or missing, especially folate, homocysteine builds up and becomes toxic to the cell. At that time, the cell is no longer able to work properly, and the inflammatory process begins.

It is known that low blood folate and a raised homocysteine concentration are associated with poor cognitive function. Researchers confirmed this information by finding that older people who had consumed the highest amounts of folate-rich foods at midlife showed significant protection from a decline in their memory and thinking skills (Luchsinger, J., et al., 2007). Vitamin B_{12} has also been studied with respect to homocysteine and Alzheimer's disease. A seven-year study of 271 Finnish people aged sixty-five to seventy-nine found that the higher their levels of B_{12}, the lower was their risk of AD, and the higher their homocysteine levels, the higher was their risk of AD (Hooshmand, B., et al., 2010).

These examples reveal just a few ways in which B vitamins are necessary for our well-being. The B vitamins are extremely important for energy generation, DNA and RNA synthesis and repair, protein and fat metabolism, red-blood cell maintenance, the preservation of healthy neurotransmitters, and more. Because of the B vitamins' complex interactions with each other and with all of the other nutrients and phytochemicals, it is essential that we include as many whole foods in our diet as possible.

The Importance of Vitamin D

The last vitamin to discuss is not really a vitamin at all, and that is vitamin D. Vitamin D is really a steroid hormone and is synthesized from cholesterol made by the liver. The process starts with the precursor vitamin D_2 that is made from cholesterol followed by the light from the sun, which converts it to vitamin D_3 in the skin. At that time, the D_3 is sent back to the liver and then onward to the kidneys to become fully active. Vitamin D_3 is also obtained from food products that are fortified with vitamin D such as cereals, orange juice, milk, and other dairy products. Other sources are eggs, beef, liver, and fatty fish or their oils—for example, the infamous cod liver oil. Vitamin D, along with calcium, has a well-established role in bone health. A growing body of evidence links its deficiency to some cancers, depression, heart disease, multiple sclerosis, type 2 diabetes, stroke, and also Alzheimer's disease and other dementias (Dickens, A., et al., 2011).

The reasons for vitamin D deficiency are multifaceted and are associated with sun exposure. Your geographic location is important; people who live in the northern regions (above the 40⁰ latitude) might miss as much as six months of vitamin D production. Working, exercising, and living predominantly indoors limit our exposure to sunlight. Sunscreens, air pollution, and clothing also reduce our sun exposure. Another reason related to seniors is that the efficiency of the skin to convert D_2 to D_3 via the sun declines with age. For all of these reasons, it is suggested that people over fifty years of age take a vitamin D_3 supplement of 600 to 1,500 IUs. An easy lab test by your doctor will reveal your vitamin D levels. If your levels are low, your doctor will put you on a regime to increase your levels safely. Research that evaluated an osteoporosis cohort study of 498 woman with the mean age of eighty found that the higher the intake of dietary vitamin D, the lower the risk of developing Alzheimer's disease (Annweiler, C., et al., 2012). These researchers acknowledged that they still do not know why vitamin D and cognitive decline are associated. One reason postulated relates to the anti-inflammatory actions of vitamin D (Krishnan and Feldman, 2011).

If you want to safely obtain vitamin D via the sun, it is suggested that sun exposure a few times a week on a sunny day will help to increase vitamin D production. Try some sunlight for ten to fifteen minutes on your face, arms, and hands in the morning before ten o'clock or in the afternoon after three o'clock—or four o'clock in the summer. Though it is still important to include a supplement if you have any of the above sun exposure issues, in accord with your doctor's recommendations.

Other Nutrients May Be Lacking

There are other nutritional deficiencies found in many patients with Alzheimer's disease. Examples are vitamin A and the carotenoids (phytochemicals related to vitamin A), as well as boron, potassium, selenium, and zinc (Balch, P., 2006). Consider taking supplements or increasing your consumption of foods that contain these important nutrients.

Take Breaks

An important idea that the Cayce readings advocated was a rest period from taking supplements. The body might begin to rely on supplements so much that it would cease to assimilate important nutrients from foods. It is the old "use it or lose it" idea. There are many ways to accomplish this rest period. On weekends, for example, eliminate your supplements. You may also choose to eliminate them on days when you are consuming wholesome, nutritious meals. Take them for a week and eliminate them for the next week, or take different supplements on different days. Your schedule will depend on the supplements you are taking and your specific needs and lifestyle.

Possible Herbs to Try

There are several herbs that have possible health benefits associated with Alzheimer's disease and memory improvement in general (Balch, P., 2006). The first is the herb well known for helping the memory, ginkgo biloba. Ginkgo biloba has many phytochemicals that act as antioxidants. It is known to increase blood flow to the brain, which improves mental function and memory. It is available as a liquid or a capsule supplement, and taking 50 to 100 mgs three times a day may treat early memory–related conditions associated with AD.

The herb with the common name of club moss or firmoss (*Huperzia serrata*) has an active compound called huperzine A that is known to improve memory, increase mental acuity, and help with language skills in persons with AD. The recommended dosage is 100 to 200 mcgs twice daily to receive these benefits.

Another interesting herb that has been used for centuries in India is turmeric, which comprises the main ingredient in curry powder. Turmeric has an active compound called curcumin that possesses antioxidant and anti–inflammatory properties. It inhibits the formation of the β–amyloid (Aβ) protein and helps eliminate existing Aβ plaques. Since the amount of curcumin in curry powder is only about 2 to 9 percent, in order to achieve its health benefits, you will need to take a supplement that contains 95 percent curcumin. It is recommended to take 400 to 600 mgs once or twice a day.

The common herbs marjoram, rosemary, oregano, parsley, thyme, the mints, and culinary sage have a phytochemical called rosmarinic acid that has the same properties as curcumin, so use them liberally in your diet. Rosemary and culinary sage have also been found to promote and enhance acetylcholine, the neurotransmitter that is found to be low in patients with Alzheimer's disease. Acetylcholine is the basis of most anti-AD drugs. Capsules containing 35 mgs of rosmarinic acid are available, with the recommended dosage of four to six capsules a day. Before taking any vitamin, mineral, or herbal supplements, first talk to your doctor or health care professional to make sure they are right for you and your particular health situation.

Points to remember for this chapter:

1. Consume more whole foods to receive the synergistic benefits of phytochemicals and vitamins, especially the B vitamins.
2. Consume more foods that are rich in vitamins C, E, and selenium.
3. Consider taking the following supplements: *methyl*cobalamin B$_{12}$, B-complex, Ester-C, a mixed tocopherol E, alpha lipoic acid, and Co-Q10.
4. Avoid antacids and take digestive enzymes instead.
5. Take a vitamin D$_3$ supplement, and enjoy some sunshine early or late in the day.

6

Simple Changes

There are several changes you can make immediately, no matter what your age, to protect and even improve your brain and to help lower your odds of developing dementia. Of course, the earlier you adopt these changes the better, especially if you are in your midlife. A whole body of research shows that your health in midlife determines what conditions you may experience in your later years.

There is no proven prescription for preventing dementia and Alzheimer's disease (AD), because there are too many lifestyle choices made at various ages that might greatly influence the outcome of the later years. Genetic makeup has some influence as well, but for the majority of people, their genomes are not as dominating a factor as their lifestyle choices. The following simple changes will not only lower your risk of dementia, and in particular AD, but will also make you feel better overall!

Physical Activity

There is mounting evidence to show that the *most* important way to reduce the risk of Alzheimer's disease is regular aerobic exercise. This choice may be as simple as a light physical activity such as walking briskly or a moderate physical activity such as jogging, swimming, or biking. The key is to select activities that you enjoy. Engage regularly in the activities for at least thirty minutes at a time, preferably for seven days a week. The activity does not have to be the same one every day, and it may vary according to the seasons. You may enjoy hiking in the summer or snowshoeing in the winter; the goal is to choose moderately strenuous exercise that will induce the heart to work harder.

Why is some form of exercise every day essential for a healthy brain? Exercise increases blood flow to the brain. Since your brain is above your heart, the blood must work against gravity to flow there. That is why aerobic activity that stimulates the heart to pump vigorously will achieve a good flow of blood to your brain. This increased blood flow helps bring in more nutrients, phytochemicals, antioxidants, and oxygen.

Nutrients Help Us

Nutrients help to repair and rebuild the brain's neurons and all of their helper cells, including the astrocytes and microglia. Phytochemicals support a wide variety of functions in the brain. Antioxidants aid in controlling oxidation, and oxygen is needed for energy production. Good blood flow also assists in the elimination of waste products caused by normal metabolism, cellular repair, and by-products that develop from free radical activity. Remember that free radicals are generated naturally from oxygen during energy production and from external sources like air pollution, cigarettes, medications, toxins, and sunlight.

Oxidative Stress

When the brain is lacking in nutrients and phytochemicals to nourish and repair the neurons as well as antioxidants to stop free radicals from oxidizing *and* is full of waste products, normal brain functioning and repair will be hampered. Oxidative stress may then take over, and inflammation may occur as the body tries to fix the many problems caused by the oxidation. (Remember that oxidative stress means that there are not enough antioxidants to stop the free radicals.) Oxidization and inflammation may become a vicious cycle with your brain on the losing side, because inflammation also causes oxidation as part of its job.

Oxidation is fine if there are plenty of antioxidants around. If there not enough antioxidants to stop the free radicals, chain reactions of oxidation may occur. That process of oxidative stress may end up damaging the neurons, especially their long, vulnerable branches called axons. This vicious cycle will eventually lead to neuronal death.

Regular Exercise

Regular exercise has been associated with a reduction of inflammation for just this reason: more antioxidants reach the brain during exercise (Reuben, D., et al., 2003). Another study revealed that people who exercised regularly and maintained a high adherence to the Mediterranean diet, which is high in fruit, vegetables, fish, and nuts and low in meat, dairy, and processed foods, decreased their risk of AD by almost 50 percent (Scarmeas, N., et al., 2009)!

Exercise increases the body's basal metabolic rate (BMR). In this case, the word basal indicates when the body is at rest or not exerting itself. When someone who exercises regularly goes about his or her normal daily life, his metabolism will perform at a higher rate than the metabolism of someone who does not exercise. The higher the BMR, the more efficiently the body is operating. This higher BMR allows the body to experience assimilation of more nutrients and phytochemicals as well as better elimination of waste products, and we understand that assimilation and elimination are the keys to health. And as we learned from chapter one, a slow metabolic rate in the brain may cause the β–amyloid (Aβ) peptide to increase and form toxic aggregates. A slow metabolism cannot eliminate those toxins properly, so they accumulate and form the senile plaques, which are considered the culprits of Alzheimer's disease.

Regular exercise also lowers the blood glucose level, which naturally tends to rise with age and which may unwittingly lead to diabetes. Exercise improves the ability of the muscles to utilize glucose and lowers blood glucose levels as a result (Wu, W., et al., 2008). Exercise also improves the brain's plasticity by increasing mental skills, attention span, and problem solving, even when commenced later in life. One study looked at sedentary older people who started an exercise program and found that they curbed their rate of cognitive decline. The study also showed that older adults who were already physically active had a much slower rate of cognitive decline than that of their sedentary counterparts (Middleton, L., et al., 2010).

More Benefits of Exercise

Being physically active enhances your immune system by lowering the stress hormones adrenaline and cortisol. Stress hormones suppress the immune response and age the brain cells, among a host of other problems attributed to stress (Balch, P., 2006). The inborn "fight-or-flight" response was very important for our ancestors. If you are being chased by a bear, you need a great deal of energy, quickly, to run very fast. One way the body responds is by turning off the immune and digestive systems in order to conserve energy. This instinctive fight-or-flight stress response initially activates adrenaline and cortisol hormones resulting from the fear of bodily harm whenever a stressful situation is encountered—bear, or no bear!

Unfortunately, since our body does not distinguish the differences in magnitude among our stresses, the hormones are still released when we are under *any* stress. If you experience relentless stress, these hormones are being released continually, and your immune and digestive systems are regularly being suppressed, as well.

Physical activity is the body's natural way to eliminate stress hormones. In present-day terms, exercising helps to eliminate our fight-or-flight responses by maintaining physical balance. Exercise even more often if you are continually stressed in your daily life. During exercise, the brain is also stimulated to produce the good-feeling hormones called endorphins. Endorphin production was the brain's way of telling our ancestors that running away from the bear was an excellent idea! Eliminating stress before it occurs is even better for the brain as well as the immune and digestive systems. I will explain more about that subject later in this chapter.

Sleep Is Important

Exercise helps with sleeping, too. Any doctor will tell you that if you do not get enough sleep, you *will* have health issues later in life. The latest research shows that seven to nine hours of sleep are needed for optimum health since the main function of sleep is cellular repair. When you are awake, your body needs a great deal of energy just to carry out its normal metabolic functions. When you are asleep, your body is able to concentrate that energy on making major repairs. For example, your body uses your sleep time for repairing DNA, cell membranes, inflammation, or glycation (when proteins and sugars bind together). These are problems that if not repaired properly may cause neurodegeneration, which may lead to Alzheimer's disease. Dr. Vincent Fortanasce, in his book *The Anti-Alzheimer's Prescription*, even theorizes that lack of sleep might be one cause of AD.

Exercise Builds New Neurons

One final and very important reason to exercise is that it builds new neurons! The old theory was that we were born with a finite number of neurons—which were all we would ever have—so we should take good care of them. We should still take good care of our neurons; but in her book, *The Secret Life of the Grown-Up Brain*, Barbara Strauch described notable research revealing that regular exercise actually creates new neurons no matter how old we are! This information makes perfect sense. Every part of our bodies makes new cells, so why not the brain? At present, research shows that our brains are not exceptions to that rule, and exercise is one way to generate these new neurons.

Mental Exercises

Challenging mental exercises are also very important to keep the mind sharp. Challenging the brain increases the neural pathways by adding new axons from neurons to connect to other neurons. Mental exercise creates new neurons just as physical exercise does. Scientists call this process "increasing your synaptic density." The synapse is a specialized junction between two neurons where chemicals called neurotransmitters are released. Most synapses occur between the end of one neuron's axon and the cell body of another neuron. This process is how information is passed from neuron to neuron, resulting in how we think. If your brain has a high density of synapses, your brain is better at handling oxidative damage. If some of the long axons are damaged, there are still many more connections for neuron-to-neuron communication.

Research from the autopsies of elderly people has shown that some of these people had various amounts of senile plaques and fibrous tangles, with no signs of AD at their deaths. These were people who had taken on mental challenges by learning and acquiring new skills regularly throughout their lives and even during their later years (Wilson, R., et al., 2007). Solving daily crossword or sudoku puzzles stimulates your brain, but to increase your synaptic density, you need to continuously learn new things that challenge your brain. It's comparable to learning to dance without changing the steps or routine. To continue the analogy, in order to create new neurons and build new axons and synapses, you need to learn new dance steps, new dance styles, and to make every routine more mentally challenging.

The good news is that you can start increasing your synaptic density at any age. One research team studied for five years 775 older Chicagoans with the average age of eighty years. The team found that those who engaged in mental activities were 40 percent less likely to develop AD than those with little or no mental activity. All of the elders in the study showed some mental decline by the end of the five years, but the decline was less steep for the cognitively active folks. Prior mental activity such as having some college education was important, but previous learning was not helpful enough. The study found that engaging in new kinds of learning in their later years was particularly important (Wilson, R., et al., 2007). The researchers pointed out that mental activity does not prevent Alzheimer's disease, nor is AD caused by lack of mental activity; but mental activity is one part of the AD puzzle.

In another study, researchers used information from the Bronx Aging Study, which had five years of data from 488 elderly people. They found that seniors who participated in at least eleven mental activities a week took much longer for memory decline to appear than those who participated in four mental activities a week, regardless of their prior education (Hall, C., et al., 2009). Examples of the mental activities of these elders were playing board and card games, reading books and magazines, going to see plays and operas, and visiting museums. Unfortunately for the couch potatoes, watching television for more than seven hours a day was linked to a higher chance of memory loss.

In Dr. Richard Restak's book, *Think Smart: A Neuroscientist's Prescription for Improving Your Brain's Performance*, research is cited indicating that we can improve our intelligence over the years by stretching it. Mental stretching is what scientists call "brain plasticity." The brain responds to challenging activities in all stages of life. Simply put, as we grow older, we can become smarter. In his book, Dr. Restak includes many excellent mental exercises that help to increase the strength of memory and intelligence.

Stretch Your Brain

There are simple things that you can do to increase your synaptic density. Stretch your brain by learning how to play chess, bridge, or other challenging board and card games. Enroll in community education classes, take up knitting or quilting, or join local dance, yoga, or tai chi classes. You may want to go to plays, operas, and museums. Read books that stimulate you to think about new ideas. Even better, try new activities or learn new skills. Undertake projects such as building models from kits, arranging your photos in scrapbooks, woodworking, or improving your home. Studying different cultures is fascinating and may lead to cooking new dishes, learning about new religions or philosophies, and even traveling to experience these new cultures firsthand.

Social interactions are very important for the brain. Social interaction forces the brain to strategize, solve problems, and consider various options during conversations by utilizing and strengthening the brain's synaptic density. Exercising with others as a social activity is ideal for a healthy brain.

Gardening helps to keep the brain sharp because of the physical and mental activity required. When planning a new garden or adding to one, concentration and creativity are involved. We carefully choose seeds and plants by learning about their behavior and care, and we make decisions about the best area to place each plant for the best chance of survival. Learning and remembering the names of each plant, both their common and scientific names, serve as a helpful mental exercise.

Walking through a beautiful garden or park is relaxing and visually stimulating, along with providing an invigorating physical exercise outdoors. Singing is beneficial for the brain—memorizing the lyrics of a favorite song challenges the brain to make new connections—and music often leads to happy feelings. To truly challenge our minds, we may choose to learn a new language or a new musical instrument. Who knows where new endeavors may lead!

Dancing

The above activities are useful for stretching the brain, but if you only want to do one thing, dancing is the best all-around activity for your brain. When dancing, you are physically exercising. You are increasing your coordination and balance, and both become very important as we age. You are also exercising mentally as you challenge your mind to learn new steps and routines. There are so many different kinds of dance that there is one for every preference. There is ballroom dancing, square dancing, ballet, jazz, modern, and rock and roll, to name just a few. Yoga and tai chi, which are also considered forms of dancing, have the extra benefit of increasing the body's flexibility.

Meditate for Better Brain Chemistry

Meditation is an important key to reducing stress, and it has been increasingly investigated by scientists who are interested in brain chemistry. Researchers have found that just as physical exercise increases the blood flow to the brain, so does meditation similarly help the brain, and with the added benefit of improving memory.

In a small research study, fifteen participants who were aged fifty-two to seventy-seven and all had memory problems were asked to meditate for twelve minutes every day for a period of eight weeks. They were instructed to repeat four sounds: SA, TA, NA, and MA. They first pronounced the sounds aloud for two minutes, then in a whisper for two minutes, then silently for four minutes, then back to a whisper for two minutes, and then aloud again for the last two minutes. A comparison group listened to two Mozart violin concertos for twelve minutes every day for the same eight-week period. At the start of the study, all participants took various cognitive tests and also had brain images taken to measure blood flow.

After the eight-week study period, both groups were tested again, including the brain imaging. The findings showed that in the meditation group, the areas of the brain associated with memory retrieval showed an increase of blood flow. Their general memory, attention, and cognition had significantly improved, as well. The group that listened to music did not have any significant improvement with cognition or blood flow (Newberg, A., et al., 2010). In response to this study, memory experts theorize that increased blood flow helps the brain to function better. As stated previously, increased blood flow is responsible for delivering more nutrients and phytochemicals to the brain as well as transporting more waste away from it. The scientists also concluded that meditation trains the brain to concentrate better. It is recognized that one *major* reason people forget is that they were not paying attention in the first place! Lastly, the researchers theorized that the relaxation one derives from meditation may play a role in stress reduction. Stress is known to control genes that affect aging and inflammation. In his book, *The Relaxation Revolution*, Dr. Herbert Benson states that what he calls the "relaxation response" deactivates these genes since it is the opposite of the stress response.

The Relaxation Response

Meditation is one way to evoke the relaxation response. Benson says meditation helps your mind to be more receptive in general because it gives your brain a break from everyday mindless thinking. The non-stop thinking is caused in part from constant connectivity by phone or computer. One of the popular meditation techniques is called "mindfulness meditation." During this kind of meditation, you concentrate on your breathing. You are encouraged to become mindful (not mindless) of your internal dialogue and thoughts, especially the negative thoughts, in order to change them into positive, constructive thoughts.

Why are negative thoughts bad for your brain? One reason is that negative thoughts activate those genes that generate the stress chemicals adrenaline and cortisol. These chemicals generate free radicals, suppress your immune system (which may increase inflammation), and also suppress your digestive system (which decreases the assimilation of vital nutrients). All of these actions may indirectly lead to the death of neurons. Scientists have also discovered that negative thinking and stress are detrimental to your brain because they decrease the availability of a substance called brain-derived neurotrophic factor (BDNF). This factor is responsible for the brain's ability to adapt and to increase its plasticity. Also, the less BDNF available in the brain, the more likely you are to become depressed. Recent studies have associated depression and Alzheimer's disease. In fact, one study found that the number of depressive episodes experienced earlier in life increased the risk of AD development (Aznar and Knudsen, 2010). Meditation is also known to help relieve depression and anxiety.

Emotions

Edgar Cayce recognized that emotions affect our health, even though the stress chemicals had not been identified at that time. The readings indicated that anger, fear, worry, jealousy, and similar emotions might cause poisons to be secreted from our glands, and that joy had the opposite effect. By glands he meant the endocrine system: the pituitary, thyroid, thymus, and adrenal glands, as well as the pancreas, ovaries, and testes. In one reading, he said " . . . Keep sweet. Keep friendly. Keep loving, if ye would keep young." (3420-1)

In conclusion, the more you meditate, the more you train your brain to concentrate and focus. The more relaxed you become, the more you remember, and the happier you become, the less inflammation you have and the healthier your brain becomes! So, how do you get started?

Meditation

Meditation is essentially a cessation of thinking—it allows the mind to be still of normal thoughts. There are many different methods and techniques, so research and experiment to find out which one is best for you and your lifestyle. The basic process is to spend ten to twenty minutes in a quiet place relaxing the body, stopping the everyday thoughts, and concentrating on the breath. You may focus on a word or a phrase while allowing silence between the repetitions. If your mind wanders, bring it back to your breath, and start again with the word or phrase. Meditation is easy to learn, it is free, and there are no adverse side effects. Meditation is also useful for children to help them focus their attention. Meditating with a child will benefit both of you.

If you have a hectic lifestyle and cannot find the time, much less a quiet spot, to meditate, begin with a five-minute meditation. All that is required is to relax your entire body and allow your thoughts to evaporate. The idea behind the five-minute meditation is to refrain from thinking for a short period of time to allow your brain to relax and recharge. Start by tensing and then relaxing your toes and feet. Then tense and relax your calves, progressing up the body until you reach your head. Now, just relax your whole body and quiet your mind for a few minutes. If thoughts arise, concentrate on your breathing, a word, or a phrase. Meditation can be done before you awake or after you go to bed. If you wake up in the middle of the night for some reason, and especially if you are worrying about the future, meditation will calm you down and help you go back to sleep. Over time, you may choose to increase your meditation time to ten and then to twenty minutes, especially when you begin to notice the benefits. Regular meditators have observed that when they have not been able to meditate for some reason, they appreciate even more the calming effect that meditation normally provides for them.

After six to eight weeks of meditation practice, your mind should be trained enough for you to summon the relaxation response under any stressful condition. This skill will turn off your stress response, especially if the stress reaction is caught right away. Gradually, stress will happen rarely in your life. Begin by taking a few deep breaths, relaxing your body, and emptying your mind. In particular, eliminate all negative thoughts that might initiate a stress response, and then focus on the problem or situation that is causing the stress. Amazing results will happen, and your brain will benefit through better brain chemistry!

Fruit for Breakfast, Lunch, or Dinner

Fruit is brain food at its best! Raw fruits contain the natural sugar, fructose (not to be associated with high fructose corn sugar). Fructose is bound to valuable nutrients, fiber, and phytochemicals so that it will not raise your blood sugar or add pounds to your waistline. Fruit should be the first thing you eat in the morning while your stomach is empty. It has unique digestive enzymes that may become diluted if there are other kinds of foods in your stomach that require different enzymes. Fruit excels in digesting fast and easily in your stomach so that the components, and especially the fructose that is readily converted to glucose, travel directly to the brain to get you started for the day. If you feel that you need more than fruit for your breakfast, wait half an hour or more to let the fruit fully digest before consuming another food such as some type of protein or carbohydrate. The exceptions are apples and bananas, which take an hour to thoroughly digest. The same waiting period applies if you consume fruit as a snack during the day.

Edgar Cayce also advocated eating fruit for breakfast, " . . . to preserve and maintain a balance: Mornings . . . Fruits . . . not as a conglomerate mass, not as combining cereals at the same meal with fruits—for these then defeat their purposes . . . " (1662-1) Your breakfast may be as simple as an apple or a melon, or it may be as festive as a fruit salad. One caveat of the Cayce readings was *not* to have citrus or citrus fruit juices with cereal and milk at the same time, choosing either cereals or fruit. It is acceptable to have some fruit and then to have some cereal and milk after waiting half an hour or more. While we are on the subject of citrus, contrary to most people's thinking, citrus fruits such as oranges, grapefruit, limes, and lemons do not increase your blood's acidic balance because almost all fruit becomes alkaline when fully digested.

The Cayce readings also had ideas about what to eat for lunch and dinner. "Noon—preferably a fresh green vegetable salad; as tomatoes, celery, lettuce, peppers, radishes, carrots, and the like. These should be grated together or chopped very fine. An oil salad dressing may be used. Evenings—a general vegetable diet, well balanced with three vegetables above the ground to one grown below . . . And the meats should only include lamb, fowl or fish . . . " (549-1)

The readings also recommended eating a fruit salad or soup for lunch or dinner and advised against consuming fried foods. We need to change the idea of meat as the main event for dinner. Vegetables should take the lead and the meat should be their small sidekick, if at all.

Alkalize Your System

Another trailblazing recommendation from the Cayce readings is the idea of keeping the pH of the body slightly alkaline by consuming a diet of 80 percent alkaline–forming foods and 20 percent acid–forming foods, which maintains the blood at a perfect pH value of 7.4. Basically, most fruits and vegetables are alkaline-forming and all meats and most grains, fats, nuts, and dairy products are acid-forming. It is more complicated, however. In her book, *Nourishing the Body Temple*, Simone Gabbay explains the concept in detail and provides an acid- and alkaline-forming food chart. Maintaining an alkaline pH between 7.35 and 7.45 is how the body operates best. All of the body's biochemical reactions, cellular enzyme reactions, assimilation, and elimination—as well as the immune system—perform optimally at this pH level. That alkaline level is not true for the stomach, which needs an acidic environment for digestion.

A pH value of seven is neutral, and below seven is considered acidic. An acidic pH slows down all of the complicated interactions the body must perform, gradually and slowly causing metabolic mayhem for all bodily functions, including the brain. A person who consumes a typical American diet will have a pH of approximately 6.5, and a person who consumes a vegan diet (consisting of no animal products) will have a pH of approximately 7.45. Depending on the intake of fruits and vegetables, everyone else is somewhere in between, excluding major health issues. Therefore, consume fresh fruit the first thing in the morning and for snacks or dinner, and consider eating vegetables as a major part of your lunch and dinner to help your body to function at its best. If you want to check your progress or are curious about your body's pH value, you can easily test it yourself with pH test strips found in health food stores. It is best to perform the test in the morning when you awake and before you drink anything, even water. Test again during the day, two hours after you put any food or liquid in your mouth, for confirmation. Simply put a small strip of the test paper in your month for a few seconds until it becomes wet. The paper will change color depending on your pH level. The pH test strips come with a color–coded scale to determine your pH.

Buy Organic

Try to purchase organic fruits and vegetables, even though it might cost a little more. Pesticides are used on non–organic crops, sometimes applied as frequently as ten times from seed to harvest. Choosing organic produce is especially important for all fruits and vegetables that blemish easily or do not have protective skins, with the most contaminated being apples, bell peppers, cherries, grapes, green beans, nectarines, pears, peaches, and strawberries. Purchasing organic foods also helps organic farmers because of the increased demand for their products. Increased demand will entice other farmers to choose organic methods, thus ending the unwholesome dependence on pesticides and synthetic fertilizers. Organic food will make both you and the planet healthier.

Drink Water

Another tip from Edgar Cayce is to drink a glass of tepid to warm water every morning upon rising or shortly afterward. The water helps flush out the waste products and toxins that have accumulated from your body's overnight repairs. The readings also advocated drinking at least six to eight glasses of tepid water daily to help continually flush the kidneys and to ensure proper eliminations. This recommendation does not apply to six to eight cups of coffee, tea, or soda. Unfortunately, the water in those drinks is bound to the ingredients in the beverages and not available for use in the body. It is best to avoid ice-cold water or beverages immediately before, during, or after a meal since very cold liquids will solidify any oily material in your stomach. This solidification will slow down digestion of the food in your stomach and may cause the entire mass of food to spoil before it is digested completely. This putrefaction may also inhibit the assimilation of nutrients and phytochemicals.

Avoid Aluminum

Aluminum has been implicated in Alzheimer's disease, not as a cause but as a contributor to the disease. One of the things the β-amyloid protein does is aggregate together, as mentioned in the first chapter. Currently, researchers think the reason for this aggregation is so that metals can stick to them. The β-amyloid with the metals can then be taken out of the brain and eliminated (Lee, H., et al., 2007). This mechanism becomes less efficient as we age, and as a consequence, aluminum is found in high concentrations in the senile plaques. A new study shows that aluminum also sticks to tau, the protein that binds to and supports the microtubule assembly. Researchers have found aggregates of aluminum and hyperphosphorylated tau, which is evidence that supports a role for aluminum in the formation of the neurofibrillary tangles (Walton, J., 2010).

Where does all of this aluminum in our bodies originate? Surprisingly, aluminum is derived from many sources. It is found naturally in air, water, and soil and is therefore found in nearly all food and water. It is also used in cookware, cooking utensils, and aluminum foil. There are many products we use every day that contain aluminum such as certain antiperspirants, toothpaste, and table salt. It is in over-the-counter antacids, painkillers, anti–inflammatory medicines, and douche preparations. Aluminum is in baking powders, bleached white flour, grated cheese, and soda pop and beer that are packed in aluminum cans. It is used in food processing, as well (Balch, P., 2006).

At present, there are many available products that will limit your exposure to aluminum. Purchase a water filter that removes the aluminum and other metals, along with chlorine, from your drinking water. Parchment paper, a product Cayce suggested for cooking, may be used instead of aluminum foil. You may choose to wrap the food in parchment paper first, and then wrap it in foil for grilling or baking. Health food stores carry antiperspirants, toothpaste, douche preparations, baking powders, and sea salt that do not contain aluminum. Do not use bleached flour, limit the amount of processed food you eat, grate your own cheese, drink filtered water instead of soft drinks, and drink beer from a bottle. Throw away any cookware made of aluminum and buy stainless steel cookware instead. Use stainless steel and wooden cooking utensils. Limit the use of painkillers and anti-inflammatory medicines, and use digestive enzymes and Slippery Elm lozenges instead of antacids. An excellent alternative to anti-inflammatory medicines is a product called Zyflamend®, produced by the company NewChapter®. Like aspirin, ibuprofen, and Celebrex®, Zyflamend is an anti-COX-2 inhibitor; but unlike aspirin and ibuprofen, it does not inhibit COX-1, making it is safer for your stomach. Zyflamend is made from a variety of herbs and phytochemicals extracted and blended in correct proportions. It comes in a daytime and nighttime formula and is found in most health food stores.

Detoxify Your System

How can you eliminate the excess aluminum and other heavy metals that might be present in your body and brain before they attach to the β–amyloid or the tau proteins? An excellent way is to use a detoxification or "detox" diet. Recommended by the Cayce readings, one of the easiest detox diets is the three-day apple fast. Apples were suggested because of their excellent cleansing effects. Apples are full of phytochemicals, especially quercetin, which is important for Alzheimer's disease. Quercetin has been shown to protect brain cells from free radicals (Tedeschi, A., et al., 2010). The best apple to use is the Red Delicious because it has more antioxidant phytochemicals than any other apple (Tsao, R., et al., 2005). Edgar Cayce suggested using Red Delicious, Arkansas Black, and Jonathan apples, and those are basically red apples as opposed to green or yellow ones. Eat as many apples as you like and drink lots of water. Coffee and tea are acceptable as long as they do not contain milk, cream, or sugar. Then, on the evening of the third day, consume one tablespoon of extra virgin olive oil. The Cayce readings suggested that the olive oil would balance the glands. Finally, how do you eliminate the β-amyloid and tau aggregates once they have formed? Remember that exercise will increase the metabolic rate of your body and the blood flow of your brain to improve the elimination of all waste products.

How to Keep It Simple

Keep things simple and always talk to your doctor before starting any new health regimen. If you do not yet have an exercise routine, begin slowly by exercising ten to fifteen minutes a few times a week, and then gradually increase your exercise time to desirable levels. If you do not have time for an exercise program, there are many small things you can do to include exercise during the day. Some examples are to park your car far away from your destination so that you have to walk to the entrance. Or use the stairs instead of the elevator even if you walk up only several flights before using the elevator for the rest. If you have to wait for someone such as a child at a music lesson or athletic practice, go for a short walk during that time. Eat lunch close to your work and walk there. When shopping in a mall, walk around the entire mall—several times if possible.

Edgar Cayce suggested taking a walk after dinner to aid digestion, and walking is a delightful way to explore your neighborhood and meet your neighbors. Get a dog; there are dozens of health attributes other than exercise that accompany owning a dog. Dogs offer love and affection, relieve stress by keeping your immune system strong, benefit your heart by lowering blood pressure, improve your social life, alleviate loneliness and depression, motivate you to exercise, and simply make you happier! There are many Web sites to help you choose a dog that is appropriate for your lifestyle. If you do not want to raise a puppy, there are plenty of adult dogs at animal shelters in need of love and companionship. When you notice the health benefits from these small steps, you may become more motivated to maintain a daily exercise routine.

Other Simple Ideas

Keep a glass of water next to your bed to drink as soon as you awake or to remind you to microwave it to a tepid temperature before drinking. Enjoy several cups of coffee or tea while you are getting ready in the morning. If you currently drink coffee with milk, cream, or sugar, drink black coffee for a week and you will never turn back. If you find the taste of black coffee too bitter, then it is too strong. Use less coffee when you brew the next pot. The nice thing about drinking coffee black is that you can taste it and realize the difference between, for example, a French roast and a Columbian roast. With so many different kinds of coffee available, you can experiment to find your favorite types. If you drink tea with milk or cream, try it with just honey, instead. If you find green tea to be too bitter, try jasmine green tea. It is much smoother and tastes delicious.

Keep a bowl of fruit on your kitchen counter so that you will choose a piece of fruit to eat as you are getting ready for your day or as you drive to work or the gym. Purchase a water filter to produce your own purified water. Carry your water in a reusable container so that you do not add plastic bottles to the landfills. Consume a large variety of salads and soups to incorporate more whole foods into your diet and to keep your blood pH slightly alkaline.

Pre-Sleep Affirmations

Another idea from the Cayce readings was the use of pre-sleep affirmations to improve many aspects of your life. As you are falling asleep, your mind is naturally relaxed and open to suggestions. This openness is the reason that watching television while going to sleep is bad for your brain. For example, watching the news may leave your brain open to negative suggestions that might influence your thoughts and brain chemistry. A recent study had subjects listen to two differ-ent musical tunes while awake, and then the researchers played back only one of the tunes while the subjects took a nap. Surprisingly, all the subjects remembered the tune they heard while napping and awake better than the tune they heard while only awake (Hildreth, Van Pelt, and Schwartz, 2012).

Since this study shows that the mind is susceptible to outside influences as we sleep, making negative or positive pre-sleep suggestions can affect us. The easiest method is to repeat positive affirmations related to your health to yourself as you fall asleep. Another technique is to customize a recording of yourself or a loved one repeating an affirmation that focuses on your health and well-being. If you have a hard time falling asleep at night without the television on, try playing some soothing music to help you relax your body and brain.

The Radiac®

Edgar Cayce's readings offered a variety of unconventional health remedies, and the Radiac® or "Impedance Device" is one of them. The Radiac was considered to be good for everyone, especially someone who was tired, inactive, or in need of increasing his or her circulation. The device was also considered useful for anyone who used the brain exceedingly. The Radiac is currently being utilized with success in the prevention of Alzheimer's disease by some people who have or have had parents with AD (EdgarCayce.org). The Radiac device may be purchased from Baar Products (Baar.com), and it is packaged with complete instructions.

My Maternal Grandparents

My grandparents who had Alzheimer's disease did not use any of these ideas, as with most people of their generation, because most of these concepts were unknown at the time. People did not commonly exercise; men worked hard at their jobs and woman worked hard doing all the housework, cooking, and child rearing. Meat and potatoes were considered good food staples, and no one knew that there were good fats and bad fats, much less trans fats. If food manufacturers made a processed, refined food product, people assumed it was good for them. Otherwise, they reasoned, why would the government let it be produced—much less sold—to the public? White flour, white sugar, and white rice were considered to be superior to their brown counterparts because they tasted purer. People in most areas of the country could not obtain fresh foods unless they had a garden. Since gardening only took place in the summertime, canned fruit and vegetables were considered a good alternative. Supplements were not widely available and were very expensive. My grandparents did not have any hobbies. I never saw them read a book or play cards or board games, although they did read the newspaper. They always had small dogs, which they walked infrequently. They were not religious and had no social life. They never traveled (except occasionally by car to visit other relatives) or went to plays, operas, or museums. My grandparents were in their early twenties during the Great Depression, so as they aged, they considered many kinds of activities to be frivolous. It cannot be claimed that any of these factors caused their Alzheimer's disease because scientists still do not know exactly what causes it. Nevertheless, the research shows that there are many facets to this disease, including multiple contributing factors, as this book implies.

My Paternal Grandmother

Even though this is anecdotal evidence, my other grandmother did not have AD when she died of pneumonia at ninety-eight years of age. She walked everywhere she went because she refused to drive a car. That idea was brought about by an accident she had the first and last time she drove a car. She went to church every Sunday, which was her social life, and prayed every day, which could be considered a type of meditation. She cooked everything from scratch and refused to eat processed, refined foods other than chocolate, which she loved! She lived on a farm as a child and then moved to my grandfather's farm when they were married. Unfortunately, he passed away when she was in her late forties, causing her to move to town. Thus, from childhood to midlife, she ate free range, pasture-fed meat, chicken, eggs, milk, and cheese. She maintained a garden until she was in her eighties, and when she had extra vegetables, she canned them in mason jars to use during the winter. Her hobby was to crochet and knit, which she did frequently. My grandmother crocheted or knitted everything from tablecloths to hats and sweaters. She even made crocheted bedspreads and blankets. Occasionally, she also made quilts for gifts. She loved to go to a variety of museums, and when our family lived in

California, my grandmother always accompanied us when we traveled to see the various historic missions. My grandmother had a closet in her house that was full of games and toys for her grandchildren, and she played these games with us, as well.

As I stated previously, these examples might not be why my paternal grandmother did not have Alzheimer's disease, but it is interesting to note the difference between the dissimilar outcomes for my grandparents in light of their lifestyle choices. The first two grandparents started showing many signs of AD in their early eighties, but my paternal grandmother was busy and active her whole life, showing no signs of dementia at her death. My mother and uncle, whose parents were the first two grandparents, are currently doing everything possible to avoid this dreaded disease. They do not follow all of the suggestions that are outlined in this book, but they have changed their eating habits for the better, quit smoking, and taken the supplements I have suggested for them. They walk their dogs every day, are avid readers, and love playing cards, board games, and computer games. They started making these changes about ten years ago when they were in their mid-sixties as I was doing the research on Alzheimer's disease for my PhD. My mother and uncle are currently in their mid-seventies and show no signs of AD. Both have had heart problems and high blood sugar levels for the past fifteen years and take various medications for those conditions.

If you are in your midlife, start *now*, and take control of your health. Incorporate into your life as many of the recommendations that are outlined in this book as possible. Take steps to avoid heart disease and diabetes, which are high risk factors for AD. If you currently have heart problems or type 2 diabetes, get them under control by following your doctor's advice. If you are in your seventies or older, don't give up; you can still change your course, as numerous studies have proven. It is never too late to initiate a health-giving lifestyle. Your heart and brain will thank you, and you will lead a long and happy life in full control!

References

Annweiler, C., Y. Rolland, A.M. Schott, H. Blain, B. Vellas, F.R. Hermann, and O. Beauchet. 2012. "Higher Vitamin D Dietary Intake is Associated with Lower Risk of Alzheimer's Disease: A 7-year Follow Up." *Journal of Gerontology, Series A, Biological Science and Medical Science* 67(11): 1205–1211.

Antony, J.W., E.W. Gobel, J.K. O'Hare, P.J. Reber, and K.A. Paller. 2012. "Cued Memory Reactivation during Sleep Influences Skill Learning." *Nature Neuroscience* 15(8): 1114–1116.

Aznar, S., and G.M. Knudsen. 2010. "Depression and Alzheimer's Disease: Is Stress the Initiating Factor in a Common Neuropathological Cascade?" *Journal of Alzheimer's Disease* 23(2): 177–193.

Balch, Phyllis. 2006. *Prescription for Nutritional Healing, Fourth Edition*. New York, NY: Avery, Penguin Books.

Barberger–Gateau, P., L. Letenneur, V. Deschamps, K. Peres, J.F. Dartigues, and S. Renaul. 2002. "Fish, Meat, and the Risk of Dementia: A Cohort Study." *British Medical Journal* 3256: 932–933.

Beauchamp, G.K., R.S. Keast, D. Morel, J. Lin, Q. Pika, C.H. Lee, A.B. Smith, and P.A. Breslin. 2005. "Phytochemistry: Ibuprofen–Like Activity in Extra–Virgin Olive Oil." *Nature* 437(7055): 45–46.

Benson, Herbert, and William Proctor. 2010. *The Relaxation Revolution*. New York, NY: Simon & Scribner.

Berenson, G.S., S.R. Srinivasan, W. Bao, W.P. Newman, R.E. Tracy, and W.A. Wattigney. 1998. "Association between Multiple Cardiovascular Risk Factors and Atherosclerosis in Children and Young Adults." *New England Journal of Medicine* 338: 1650–1656.

Bonda, D.J., X. Wang, G. Perry, A. Nunomura, M Tabaton, and X. Zhu. 2010. "Oxidative Stress in Alzheimer Disease: A Possibility for Prevention." *Neuropharmacology* 59(4–5): 290–294.

Boustani, M., K.S. Hall, K.A. Lane, H. Aljadhey. S. Gao, F. Unverzagt, M.D. Murray, A. Ogunniyi, and H. Hendrie. 2007. "The Association between Cognition and Histamine–2 Receptor Antagonist in African Americans." *Journal of the Geriatric Society* 55(8): 1248–1253.

Castellani, R.J., A. Nunomura, H.G. Lee, G. Perry, and M.A. Smith. 2008. "Phosphorylated Tau: Toxic, Protective, or None of the Above." *Journal of Alzheimer's Disease* 14(4): 1377–1383.

Commenges, D., V. Scotet, S. Renaud, H. Jacqmin–Gadda, P. Barberger–Gateau, and J.F. Dartigues. 2000. "Intake of Flavonoids and the Risk of Dementia." *European Journal of Epidemiology* 16(4): 357–363.

Cordy, J.M., N.M. Hooper, and A.J. Turner. 2006. "The Involvement of Lipid Rafts in Alzheimer's Disease." *Molecular Membrane Biology* 23: 111–122.

Das, U.N. 2008. "Folic Acid and Polyunsaturated Fatty Acids Improve Cognitive Function and Prevent Depression, Dementia, and Alzheimer's Disease—But How and Why?" *Prostaglandins, Leukotrienes and Essential Fatty Acids* 78(1): 11–19.

Deschamps, V., P. Barberger–Gateau, E. Peuchant, and J.M. Orgogozo. 2001. "Nutritional Factors in Cerebral Aging and Dementia: Epidemiological Arguments for a Role of Oxidative Stress." *Neuroepidemiology* 20: 7–15.

Dickens, A.P., I.A. Lang, K.M. Langa, K. Kos, and D.J. Llewellyn. 2010. "Vitamin D, Cognitive Dysfunction, and Dementia in Older Adults." *CNS Drugs* 25(8): 626–639.

Erasmus, Udo. 1993. *Fats that Heal, Fats that Kill: The Complete Guide to Fats, Oils, Cholesterol, and Human Health.* Vancouver, Canada: Alive Books.

Eskelinen, M.H., T. Ngandu, J. Tuomilehtso, H. Soininen, and M. Kivipelto. 2009. "Midlife Coffee and Tea Drinking and the Risk of Late–Life Dementia: A Population Based CAIDE Study." *Journal of Alzheimer's Disease* 16: 85–91.

Farris, W., S. Mansourian, Y. Chan, L. Lindsley, E.A. Eckman, M.P. Frosch, C.B. Eckman, C.B. Tanzi, D.J. Selkoe, and S. Guenett. 2003. "Insulin–Degrading Enzyme Regulates the Levels of Insulin, Amyloid β–Protein, and the β–Amyloid Precursor Protein Intracellular Domain *in vivo.*" *Protocols of the National Academy of Science USA* 100(7): 4162–4167.

Fiala, M, J. Lin, J. Ringman, V. Kemani–Arab, G. Tsao, A. Patel, A.S. Lossinsky, M.C. Graves, A. Gustavson, J. Sayre, E. Sofroni, T. Suarez, F. Chiappelli, and G. Bernard. 2005. "Ineffective Phagocytosis of Amy-loid–Beta by Macrophages of Alzheimer's Disease Patients." *Journal of Alzheimer's Disease* 7(3): 221–232.

Fortanasce, Vincent. 2008. *The Anti-Alzheimer's Prescription: The Science-Proven Plan to Start at Any Age.* New York: Gotham Books.

Freund–Levi, Y., M. Eriksdotter–Jönhagen, T. Cederholm, H. Basun, G. Faxén–Irving, A. Garlind, I. Vedi, B. Vessby, L.O. Wahlund, and J. Palmblad. 2006. "ω–3 Fatty Acids Treatment in 174 Patients with Mild to Moderate Alzheimer's Disease: Omega AD Study." *Archives of Neurology* 63: 1402–1408.

Galli, C., and F. Marangoni. 2006. "N–3 Fatty Acids in the Mediterranean Diet." *Prostaglandins, Leukotrienes, and Essential Fatty Acids* 75(3): 129–133.

Gamba, P., G. Leonarduzzi, E. Tamagno, M. Guglielmotto, G. Testa, B. Sottero, S. Gargiulo, F. Biasi, A. Mauro, J. Vina, and G. Poli. 2011. "Interaction Between 24–Hydroxycholesterol, Oxidative Stress, and Amyloid-β in Amplifying Neuronal Damage in Alzheimer's Disease: Three Partners in Crime." *Aging Cell* 10(3): 403–417.

Green, K.N., J.S. Steffan, H. Martinez–Coria, X. Sun, S.S. Schreiber, L.M. Thompson, and F.M. LaFerla. 2008. "Nicotinamide Restores Cognition in Alzheimer's Disease Transgenic Mice Via a Mechanism Involving Sirtuin Inhibition and Selective Reduction of Thr231-Phosphotau." *Journal of Neuroscience* 28(45): 11500–11510.

Halpern, George. 2001. *Lyprinol: A Natural Solution for Arthritis and Other Inflammatory Disorders.* New York: Penguin/Putnam/Avery.

Hall, C.B., R.B. Lipton, M. Sliwinski, M.J. Katz, C.A. Derby, and J. Verghese. 2009. "Cognitive Activities Delay Onset of Memory Decline in Persons Who Develop Dementia." *Neurology* 73(5): 356–361.

Hardy, J., and D.J. Selkoe. 2002. "The Amyloid Hypothesis of Alzheimer's

Disease: Progress and Problems on the Road to Therapeutics." *Science* 297: 353–356.

Hildreth, K.L., R.E. Van Pelt, and R.S. Schwartz. 2012. "Obesity, Insulin Resistance, and Alzheimer's Disease." *Obesity (Silver Springs)* 20(8): 1549–1557.

Hooshmand, B., A. Solomon, I. Kareholt, J. Leiviska, M. Rusanen, S. Ahtiluto, B. Winblad, T. Laatikainen, H. Soininen, and M. Kivipelto. 2010. "Homocysteine and Holostranscoblamin and the Risk of Alzheimer Disease: A Longitudinal Study." *Neurology* 75(16): 1408–1414.

Kalmijn, S., P.J. Van Boxtel, M. Ocke, W. Verschuren, D. Kromjout, and I.J. Launer. 2004. "Dietary Intake of Fatty Acids and Fish in Relation to Cognitive Performance at Middle Age." *Neurology* 62: 275–280.

Krishnan, A.V., and D. Feldman. 2011. "Mechanisms of the Anti-Cancer and Anti-Inflammatory Actions of Vitamin D." *Annual Review of Pharmacology and Toxicology* 51: 311–336.

Jensen, Bernard, and Mark Anderson. 1990. *Empty Harvest: Understanding the Link between Our Food, Our Immunity and Our Planet.* Garden City Park, New York: Avery Publishing Group Inc.

Lee, H., X. Zhu, R.J. Castellani, A. Nunomura, G. Perry, and M.A. Smith. 2007. "Amyloid-β in Alzheimer Disease: The Null Versus the Alternate Hypotheses." *Journal of Pharmacology and Experimental Therapeutics* 321: 823–829.

Luchsinger, J.A., M.X. Tang, J. Miller, R. Green, and R. Mayeux. 2007. "Relation of Higher Folate Intake to Lower Risk of Alzheimer's Disease in the Elderly." *Archives of Neurology* 64(1): 86–92.

Mangialasche, F., M. Kivipelto, P. Mecocci, D. Rizzuto, K. Palmer, B. Winblad, and L. Fratiglioni. 2010. "High Plasma Levels of Vitamin E Forms and Reduced Alzheimer's Disease Risk in Advanced Age." *Journal of Alzheimer's Disease* 20(4): 1029–1037.

Martin, A., J.A. Joseph, and A.M. Cuervo. 2002. "Stimulatory Effect of Vitamin C on Autophagy in Glial Cells." *Journal of Neurochemistry* 82: 538–549.

McDonald, S.R., R.S. Sohal, and M.J. Forster. 2005. "Concurrent Administration of Coenzyme Q10 and Alpha-Tocopherol Improves Learning in Aged Mice." *Free Radical Biological Medicine* 38(6): 729–736.

Middleton, L.E., D.E. Barnes, Y. Lui, and K. Yaffe. 2010. "Physical Activity over the Life Course and Its Association with Cognitive Performance and Impairment in Old Age." *Journal of the American Geriatric Society* 58(7): 1322–1326.

Moreira, P.I., M.S. Santos, C.R. Oliveira, J.C. Shenk, M.A. Smith, X. Zhu, and G. Perry. 2008. "Alzheimer Disease and the Role of Free Radicals in the Pathogenesis of the Disease." *CNS Neurological Disorders Drug Targets* 7(1): 3–10.

Munch, G., W. Deuther-Conrad, and J. Gasic-Milenkovic. 2002. "Glycoxidative Stress Creates a Vicious Cycle of Neurodegeneration in Alzheimer's Disease—A Target for Neuroprotective Treatment Strategies?" *Journal of Neural Transmission* 62: 303–307.

Newberg, A.B., N. Wintering, D.S. Khalsa, H. Roggenkamp, and M.R. Waldman. 2010. "Meditation Effects on Cognitive Function and Cerebral Blood Flow in Subjects with Memory Loss: A Preliminary Study." *Journal of Alzheimer's Disease* 20(2): 517–526.

Papp, K.A. 2007. "The Safety of Etanercept for the Treatment of Plaque Psoriasis." *Therapeutics Clinical Risk Management* 3(2): 245–258.

Perricone, Nicolas. 2000. *The Wrinkle Cure: Unlock the Power of Cosmeceuticals for Supple, Youthful Skin.* New York: Warner Books.

Petersen, R.B., A. Nunomura, H.G. Lee, G. Casadesus, G. Perry, M.A. Smith, and X. Zhu. 2007. "Signal Transduction Cascades Associated with Oxidative Stress in Alzheimer's Disease." *Journal of Alzheimer's Disease* 11(2): 143–152.

Pettegrew, J.W., and R.J. McClure. 2002. "Acetyl-L-Carnitine as a Possible Therapy for Alzheimer's Disease." *Expert Review of Neurotherapeutics* 2(5): 647–654.

Planel, E., K. Yasutake, S.C. Fujita, and K. Ishiguro. 2001. "Inhibition of Protein Phosphatase 2A Overrides Tau Protein Kinase 1/Glycogen

Synthase 3 Beta and Cyclin-Dependent Kinase 5 Inhibition and Results in Tau Hyperphosphorylation in the Hippocampus of Starved Mice." *Journal of Biological Chemistry* 276: 34298–34306.

Pressman, Alan H., and Sheila Buff. 2007. *The Complete Idiot's Guide to Vitamins & Minerals, 3rd Edition.* New York: Alpha Books/Penguin Group.

Reitz, C., T. den Heijer, C. van Duijn, A. Hofman, and M.M. Breteler. 2007. "Relation between Smoking and Risk of Dementia and Alzheimer's Disease: The Rotterdam Study." *Neurology* 69(10): 998–1005.

Restak, Richard. 2009. *Think Smart: A Neuroscientist's Prescription for Improving Your Brain's Performance.* New York: Riverhead Books/Penguin Books.

Reuben, D.B., L. Judd-Hamilton, T.B. Harris, and T.E. Seeman. 2003. "The Associations between Physical Activity and Inflammatory Markers in High-Functioning Older Persons: MacArthur Studies of Successful Aging." *Journal of American Geriatric Society* 51(8): 1125–1130.

Riviere, S., I. Birlouez-Aragon, F. Nourhashemi, and B. Vellas. 1998. "Low Plasma Vitamin C in Alzheimer Patients despite an Adequate Diet." *International Journal of Geriatric Psychiatry* 13: 749–754.

Sanchez-Moreno, C., and A. Martin. 2006. "Protective Effect of Vitamin C against Protein Modification in the Brain: Its Importance to Neurodegenerative Conditions." In: *Focus on Nutritional Research*, edited by Tony P. Starks, 33–48. Hauppauge, NY: Nova Science Publishers.

Scarmeas, N., J.A. Luchsinger, N. Schupf, A.M. Brickman, S. Cosentino, M.X. Tang, and Y. Stern. 2009. "Physical Activity, Diet, and Risk of Alzheimer's Disease." *Journal of the American Medical Association* 302(6): 627–637.

Scarmeas, N., Y. Stern, R. Mayeux, J.J. Manly, N. Schupf, and J.A. Luchsinger. 2009. "Mediterranean Diet and Mild Cognitive Impairment." *Archives of Neurology* 66(2): 216–225.

Sen, C.K., S. Khanna, and S. Roy. 2006. "Tocotrienol: The Natural Vitamin E to Defend the Nervous System?" *Annals of the New York Academy of Sciences* 1031: 127–142.

Snowdon, D.A., C.L. Tully, C.D. Smith, K.P. Riley, and W.R. Markesbery. 2000. "Serum Folate and the Severity of Atrophy of the Neocortex in Alzheimer's Disease: Findings from the Nun Study." *American Journal of Clinical Nutrition* 71: 933–938.

Strauch, Barbara. 2011. *The Secret Life of the Grown-up Brain: The Surprising Talents of the Middle-Aged Mind.* New York: Penguin Group, Inc.

Struble, R.G., T. Ala, P.R. Patrylo, G.J. Brewer, and X. Yan. 2010. "Is Brain Amyloid Production a Cause or a Result of Dementia of the Alzheimer Type?" *Journal of Alzheimer's Disease* 22(2): 393–399.

Su, B., X. Wang, A. Nunomura, P.I. Moreira, H.G. Lee, G. Perry, M.A. Smith, and X. Zhu. 2008. "Oxidative Stress Signaling in Alzheimer's Disease." *Current Alzheimer's Research* 5(6): 525–532.

Sultana, R., M. Perluigi, and D.A. Butterfield. 2006. "Postmortem Analysis of Alzheimer's Disease Brain Shows Elevated Markers of Oxidative Stress, Protein, and Lipid Oxidation Products." *Antioxidant and Redox Signaling* 8(11–12): 2020–2037.

Tedeschi, A., G. D'Errico, M.R. Lauro, F. Sansone, S. Di Marino, A.M. D'Ursi, and R.P. Aquino. 2010. "Effects of Flavonoids on the Abeta (25–35)–Phospholipid Bilayers Interaction." *European Journal of Medical Chemistry* 45(9): 3998–4003.

Tsao, R., R. Yang, S. Xie, E. Sockovie, and S. Khanizadeh. 2005. "Which Polyphenolic Compounds Contribute to the Total Antioxidant Activities of Apple?" *Journal of Agriculture and Food Chemistry* 53(12): 4989–4995.

Vassar, R., D.M. Kovacs, R. Yan, and P.C. Wong. 2009. "The β–Secretase Enzyme BACE in Health and Alzheimer's Disease: Regulation, Cell Biology, Function, and Therapeutic Potential." *The Journal of Neuroscience* 29(41): 12787–12794.

Walton, J.R. 2010. "Evidence for Participation of Aluminum in Neurofibrillary Tangle Formation and Growth in Alzheimer's Disease."

Journal of Alzheimer's Disease 22(1): 65–72.

Watson, G.S., E.R. Peskind, S. Asthana, K. Purganan, C. Wait, D. Chapman, M.W. Schwartz, S. Plymate, and S. Craft. 2003. "Insulin Increases CSF Aβ42 Levels in Normal Older Adults." *Neurology* 60(12): 1899–1903.

Weingartner, O., M. Bohm, and U. Laufs. 2011. "Cholesterol–Lowering Foods and the Reduction of Serum Cholesterol Levels." *Journal of the American Medical Association* 306(20): 2217–2218.

Weir, D.G. and A.M. Molloy. 2000. "Microvascular Disease and Dementia in the Elderly: Are They Related to Hyperhomocysteinemia?" *American Journal of Clinical Nutrition* 71: 859–860

Whitaker, Julian M. 2002. *Reversing Heart Disease: A Vital New Program to Help Prevent, Treat, and Eliminate Cardiac Problems without Surgery.* New York: Warner Books.

Whitbourne, Susan Krauss. 2002. *The Aging Individual: Physical and Psychological Perspectives.* 2nd ed. New York: Springer Publishing Company.

Whitmer, R., D.R. Gustafson, E. Barrett-Connor, M.N. Hann, E.P. Gunderson, and K. Yaffe. 2008. "Central Obesity and Increased Risk of Dementia More than Three Decades Later." *Neurology* 71(14): 1057–1064.

Whitney, Eleanor Noss, and Sharon Rady Rolfes. 2002. *Understanding Nutrition.* 9th ed. Belmont, CA: Wadsworth/Thomson Learning.

Wilson, R.S., P.A. Scherr, J.A. Schneider, Y. Tang, and D.A. Bennett. 2007. "Relation of Cognitive Activity to Risk of Developing Alzheimer's Disease." *Neurology* 69(20): 1911–1920.

Wu, W., A.M. Brickman, J. Luchsinger, P. Ferrazzano, P. Pichiule, M. Yoshita, T. Brown, C. DeCarli, C.A. Barnes, R. Mayeux, S.J. Vannucci, and S.A. Small. 2008. "The Brain in the Age of Old: The Hippocampal Formation is Targeted Differentially by Diseases of Late Life." *Annuals of Neurology* 64(6): 698–706.

Zandi, P.P., J.C. Anthony, A.S. Khachaturian, S.V. Stone, D. Gustafson, J.T. Tschanz, M.C. Norton, K.A. Welsh-Bohmer, and J.C. Breitner. 2004.

"Reduced Risk of Alzheimer's Disease in Users of Antioxidant Vitamin Supplements: The Cache County Study." *Archives of Neurology* 61(1): 82–88.

Zhu, X., A.K. Raina, H.G. Lee, G. Casadesus, M.A. Smith, and G. Perry. 2008. "Oxidation Stress Signaling in Alzheimer's Disease." *Brain Research* 1000(1–2): 32–39.

Resources

Baar Products, Inc.: The Official Supplier of Edgar Cayce Health Care Products, (800) 269-2502 or Baar.com. This is the supplier of the Radiac® device, along with many other products recommended by the Cayce readings.

Oils of Aloha: (800) 367-6010 or OilsofAloha.com. Hawaiian macadamia nut oil specialist. You may want to purchase the macadamia nut oil sampler to try four of their blends in one set.

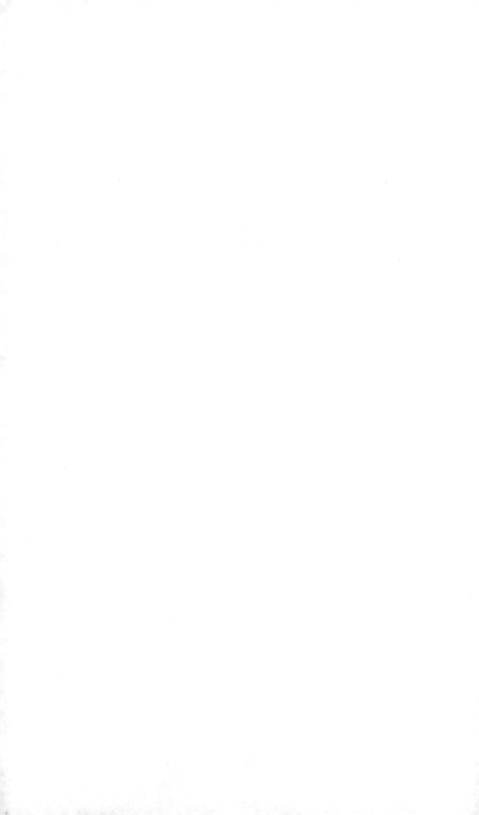

Suggested Reading

Beyond Aspirin: Nature's Answer to Arthritis, Cancer & Alzheimer's Disease by Thomas M. Newmark and Paul Schulick. Prescott, AZ: Hohm Press, 2000. This book explains the inflammation–causing enzyme known as "COX-2" and gives information on natural ways to control inflammation.

Change Your Brain, Change Your Life and *Change Your Brain, Change Your Body* by Daniel G. Amen, MD. New York: Crown Publishing Group, 1998 and 2010. Dr. Amen is a neuroscientist and an expert on the relationship of the brain, behavior, and biochemistry. He reveals ways you can change how your brain operates through simple, self–administered "brain prescriptions" to heal your body and your life.

Fats that Heal, Fats that Kill by Udo Erasmus. Burnaby, BC Canada: Alive Books, 1993. This book is a comprehensive guide to fats, oils and cholesterol related to human health.

Mindfulness: an Eight-Week Plan for Finding Peace in a Frantic World by Mark Williams and Danny Penman. Emmaus, PA: Rodale Press, Inc., 2011. The authors offer a set of simple practices designed for a busy lifestyle to help people obtain the benefits of meditation.

Nourishing the Body Temple by Simone Gabbay. Virginia Beach, VA: A.R.E. Press, 1999 (out of print but available for Kindle). A nutritional approach based on the dietary wisdom of Edgar Cayce is suggested.

Nourishing Traditions by Sally Fallon with Mary G. Enig, PhD. Washington, DC: New Trends Publishing, Inc., 2001. This book is a cookbook with recipes that explores the culinary customs of our ancestors. It challenges our current, politically correct diet that has increased chronic diseases that were unheard of in our ancestors' time.

Nutrition and Physical Degeneration by Weston A. Price, DDS. New Canaan, CT: Keats Publishing, Inc., 1989 (first published in 1939). A fascinating comparison of native and modern diets and their effects on health is offered, along with an abundance of pictures to back up the findings.

Prescription for Nutritional Healing, Fifth Edition by Phyllis A. Balch, CNC. NY: Avery Trade, 2010. This book is an invaluable reference guide to natural health, providing an abundance of information from general holistic health to combating specific conditions naturally.

The Secret Life of the Grown-up Brain by Barbara Strauch. NY: Penguin Books, 2011. Barbara Strauch explores the latest research that finds the middle-aged brain to be far more flexible than previously assumed, and surprisingly more talented.

4TH DIMENSION PRESS

An Imprint of A.R.E. Press

4th Dimension Press is an imprint of A.R.E. Press, the publishing division of Edgar Cayce's Association for Research and Enlightenment (A.R.E.).

We publish books, DVDs, and CDs in the fields of intuition, psychic abilities, ancient mysteries, philosophy, comparative religious studies, personal and spiritual development, and holistic health.

For more information, or to receive a catalog, contact us by mail, phone, or online at:

4th Dimension Press
215 67th Street
Virginia Beach, VA 23451-2061
800-333-4499

4THDIMENSIONPRESS.COM

Who Was Edgar Cayce?
Twentieth Century Psychic and Medical Clairvoyant

Edgar Cayce (pronounced Kay-Cee, 1877-1945) has been called the "sleeping prophet," the "father of holistic medicine," and the most-documented psychic of the 20th century. For more than 40 years of his adult life, Cayce gave psychic "readings" to thousands of seekers while in an unconscious state, diagnosing illnesses and revealing lives lived in the past and prophecies yet to come. But who, exactly, was Edgar Cayce?

Cayce was born on a farm in Hopkinsville, Kentucky, in 1877, and his psychic abilities began to appear as early as his childhood. He was able to see and talk to his late grandfather's spirit, and often played with "imaginary friends" whom he said were spirits on the other side. He also displayed an uncanny ability to memorize the pages of a book simply by sleeping on it. These gifts labeled the young Cayce as strange, but all Cayce really wanted was to help others, especially children.

Later in life, Cayce would find that he had the ability to put himself into a sleep-like state by lying down on a couch, closing his eyes, and folding his hands over his stomach. In this state of relaxation and meditation, he was able to place his mind in contact with all time and space—the universal consciousness, also known as the super-conscious mind. From there, he could respond to questions as broad as, "What are the secrets of the universe?" and "What is my purpose in life?" to as specific as, "What can I do to help my arthritis?" and "How were the pyramids of Egypt built?" His responses to these questions came to be called "readings," and their insights offer practical help and advice to individuals even today.

The majority of Edgar Cayce's readings deal with holistic health and the treatment of illness. Yet, although best known for this material, the sleeping Cayce did not seem to be limited to concerns about the physical body. In fact, in their entirety, the readings discuss an astonishing 10,000 different topics. This vast array of subject matter can be narrowed down into a smaller group of topics that, when compiled together, deal with the following five categories: (1) Health-Related Information; (2) Philosophy and Reincarnation; (3) Dreams and Dream Interpretation; (4) ESP and Psychic Phenomena; and (5) Spiritual Growth, Meditation, and Prayer.

Learn more at EdgarCayce.org.

What Is A.R.E.?

Edgar Cayce founded the non-profit Association for Research and Enlightenment (A.R.E.) in 1931, to explore spirituality, holistic health, intuition, dream interpretation, psychic development, reincarnation, and ancient mysteries—all subjects that frequently came up in the more than 14,000 documented psychic readings given by Cayce.

The Mission of the A.R.E. is to help people transform their lives for the better, through research, education, and application of core concepts found in the Edgar Cayce readings and kindred materials that seek to manifest the love of God and all people and promote the purposefulness of life, the oneness of God, the spiritual nature of humankind, and the connection of body, mind, and spirit.

With an international headquarters in Virginia Beach, Va., a regional headquarters in Houston, regional representatives throughout the U.S., Edgar Cayce Centers in more than thirty countries, and individual members in more than seventy countries, the A.R.E. community is a global network of individuals.

A.R.E. conferences, international tours, camps for children and adults, regional activities, and study groups allow like-minded people to gather for educational and fellowship opportunities worldwide.

A.R.E. offers membership benefits and services that include a quarterly body-mind-spirit member magazine, *Venture Inward*, a member newsletter covering the major topics of the readings, and access to the entire set of readings in an exclusive online database.

Learn more at EdgarCayce.org.